Perioperative TOE

Perioperative TOE

Stefaan Bouchez

Transoesophageal echocardiography

ACADEMIA
PRESS

Uitgeverij Academia Press
Coupure Rechts 88
9000 Gent
België

www.academiapress.be

Uitgeverij Academia Press maakt deel uit van Lannoo Uitgeverij,
de boeken- en multimediadivisie van Uitgeverij Lannoo nv.

ISBN 978-94-014-6940-1
D/2020/45/250
NUR 876

Stefaan Bouchez
Perioperative TOE. Transoesophageal echocardiography.
Gent, Academia Press, 2023, 282 p.

Eerste druk, 2023

Vormgeving cover: Nico Goossens
Vormgeving binnenwerk: puurprint
Zetwerk binnenwerk: puurprint
Illustraties: Nico Goossens en Stefaan Bouchez

Content

Introduction

Over the last decades, the utility of perioperative echocardiography for monitoring cardiac performance and diagnosing cardiac pathology has become increasingly evident. Advanced understanding of perioperative transoesophageal echocardiography (TOE) skills next to the mounting complexity of surgical procedures and patient pathology is expected from physicians supporting perioperative patient care. At the same time, TOE knowledge has progressed with new guidelines and advanced techniques finding their place in daily clinical practice.

The authors of this booklet were eager to share their knowledge and enthusiasm to all interested practitioners of TOE. The easily approachable and well-defined text offers the clinicians a practical resource in the use of TOE for a particular clinical challenge whether performed in the operating room, structural heart and catheterization laboratory room, intensive care unit or the emergency room. The chapters have been reduced in size, focused on clinical practice, and presented in a quick reference outline format. The aim of this booklet was not only to serve as a clinical guide but also intended as a valuable aid for those who are seeking certification in TOE.

Acknowledgement is given to my friends and colleagues of EACTAIC for their contribution to this booklet. Also, I want to thank Nico Goossens for his support in creating the illustrations.

Keep challenging yourself!
September 2023
Stefaan Bouchez, MD, FASE

" The greatest value of a picture
is when it forces us to notice
what we never expected to see. **"**

John W. Tukey 1977

1

Transoesophageal Echocardiography Safety

HENRY SKINNER

1.1 Indications and contra-indications

- Transoesophageal Echocardiography (TOE) is considered a **standard of care during cardiac surgery**.
  - Europe: TOE in all adult patients undergoing cardiac or thoracic aortic surgery.
  - North America: TOE for all open-heart surgery and to be considered for CABG.
- TOE causes serious injury in <1/1000 examinations.
- TOE-related injury should inform the consent process and serve as a reminder that performing a TOE carries an inherent risk.
- No TOE means no TOE-related damage but to withhold TOE in a patient undergoing cardiac surgery may not be the patient's interest!
- Contra-indications include perforated viscus, significant oesophageal pathology (stricture, trauma, tumour, scleroderma, Mallory-Weiss tear, diverticulum), upper gastrointestinal (GI) bleeding, recent upper GI surgery and oesophagectomy, although safe TOE use in a patient with a previous oesophagectomy has been reported.
- TOE may be considered in patients with gastro-oesophageal disease if the expected benefit outweighs the potential risk, provided appropriate precautions are followed.

1.2 Incidence

There seems to be a higher incidence of injuries in cardiac theatres compared to the echolab; this is because the cardiac surgical patient (asleep and paralysed) cannot react to noxious stimuli or help to swallow the probe, they tend to have more extended examinations and are (probably) more often used for teaching.

COMPLICATION RELATED TO TOE	INCIDENCE
Sore throat	1 in 12
Swallowing dysfunction	1 in 25
Oropharyngeal mucosal injury	1 in 500
Oesophageal perforation and GI bleed	1 in 1250
Dental injury	1 in 3000
Death	1 in 3000

1.3   Mechanism of injury

- Injury follows the path of insertion of the probe all the way from the mouth (lips, teeth and tongue) to the stomach.
- Injury is caused when an excessive force (absolute or relative) is exerted on tissue during probe insertion or manipulation (especially probe flexion with the probe in the oesophagus).
- Tissue necrosis can also be caused by sustained pressure exerted by a static probe in situ.
- When acquiring a Short Axis (SAX) view of the left ventricle (LV), the tip of the probe may actually still be in the oesophagus and there is thus a clear potential for tissue trauma if the probe is ante- or retroflexed when the operator assumes the probe is already within the stomach.

1.4   Risk factors

- Risk factors associated with oesophageal injury are small patient size, female sex, advanced age, prolonged procedure, difficult probe placement, cardiomegaly, low cardiac output, MitraClip® procedure (interventional cardiology) and return to the operating room.
- Many injuries occur in the absence of known risk factors.

1.5 Oesophageal injury

- A ruptured oesophagus carries a mortality of approximately 20%.
- The hall marks of good management include a high index of suspicion, early diagnosis and early surgical intervention.
- Blood in the oropharynx or blood on removal of the TOE probe is an early clue but does not necessarily imply significant injury.
- Inability to visualize cardiac structures during the TOE examination should alert the operator to the possibility that the probe may not be within the oesophagus or stomach.
- Time to presentation is often delayed with diagnosis beyond 24h in more than half of patients.
- Signs of rupture may be subtle and frequently masked by post-operative intubation and sedation.
- Meckler's triad of vomiting, pain, subcutaneous emphysema (signs of spontaneous rupture) is seldom present and the initial chest X-ray (CXR) may be normal (33% in one study). Non-specific signs include dyspnoea, fever, bloody nasogastric (NG) aspirates.
- Literature suggests a low threshold to insert a NG tube if it was difficult to insert the probe or if blood is present on probe removal.
- A contrast oesophagography should be performed to identify the site of perforation as this determines subsequent management.

1.6 Prevention

- Insert the probe by preference with the aid of a video-laryngoscope or under direct vision with the use of a laryngoscope and generous lubrication. This markedly reduces the incidence of swallowing dysfunction and oropharyngeal mucosal injury and helps the operator to stay in the midline.

- If resistance is met, do not force insertion; ask for senior help, ensure the probe is in a neutral position, and realign the probe.
- Never insert or remove the probe in a locked position.
- Direct supervision is advised until the operator is deemed proficient.
- Limit unnecessary probe manipulation.
- If TOE is considered essential/highly desirable in patients with prior oesophageal disease risk, consider referral for an upper GI endoscopy first and consider performing a targeted rather than comprehensive examination.
- Distraction of the anaesthetist by TOE could be detrimental to performing other complex tasks that require a high level of cognitive processing and ideally time should be set aside to perform the TOE prior to commencing surgery.

1.7 References

1. Ramalingam G, et al. *Complications related to peri-operative transoesophageal echocardiography – a one-year prospective national audit by the Association of Cardiothoracic Anaesthesia and Critical Care*. Anaesthesia 2020; 75(1):21-26
2. Hilberath JN, et al. *Safety of Transesophageal Echocardiography*. J Am Soc Echocardiogr 2010; 23:1115-27.
3. Lennon MJ, et al. *Transesophageal echocardiography-related gastrointestinal complications in cardiac surgical patients*. J Cardiothorac Vasc Anesth 2005;19:141-5.

2

TOE Views & Comprehensive Exam

ECKHARD MAUERMANN
MANFRED SEEBERGER

2.1 Aims and Goals

- Goals: qualitative and quantitative assessment of morphology and function of chambers, valves and vessels.
- Aims: to guide and document interdisciplinary management AND to improve patient outcomes.

2.2 Indications

2.2.1 Cardiac and thoracic aortic procedures

- CABG: (aortic and venous cannulation, wall motion, separation from cardiopulmonary bypass (CPB) and haemodynamic management, new findings [such as patent foramen ovale (PFO)], etc.).
- Valve repair/replacement (as above + confirmation of indication, visualization of other surgical steps (e.g. peripheral cannulation, LV vent placement, LV size during cardioplegia, etc.), mechanisms of valve pathology, sizing of valve, assessment of valve repair/replacement, etc.).
- Thoracic procedures (as above + confirmation of indication, assessment of aorta (entry/exit flaps, true/false lumen, wire for direct aortic cannulation), aortic valve (AV), coronary arteries, anastomoses, and reinsertion of coronary buttons, etc.).
- Guiding interventional or non-surgical procedures (MitraClip®,
- Transapical valves, occluder devices, thrombus assessment prior to cardioversion, etc.).

2.2.2 Noncardiac surgery

- Patient risk factors (severely reduced ventricular function, valve pathologies).
- Intervention (liver surgery, thoracic surgery).
- Unexplained persistent hypotension or hypoxaemia.

- Assessment of cardiac function and tamponade.
- Assessment of mechanical support (IABP, Impella®, ECMO).

2.3   Image acquisition

2.3.1   Probe manipulation

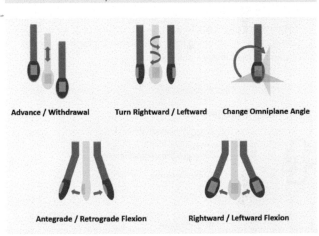

Advance / Withdrawal   Turn Rightward / Leftward   Change Omniplane Angle

Antegrade / Retrograde Flexion   Rightward / Leftward Flexion

2.3.2   General considerations of image acquisition

- Electrocardiography (ECG) for better understanding of the images (not just for ECG gating).
- Use apnoea when necessary and permissible.
- Optimize the probe to obtain the ideal acoustic window.
  - Always move the probe in only one dimension at a time.
  - Small movements of the probe result in substantial changes of the imaging plane.

- Understand ultrasound image creation and optimize what you want to see.
  - Adjust depth/use zoom/decrease width of the two-dimensional (2D) imaging sector to maximize resolution in the area of interest.
  - Move focus to the area of interest (best lateral resolution).
  - Optimize spatiotemporal resolution (narrow sector to increase frame rate, use of ECG-gating, etc.).
  - Use presets for resolution, general and penetration modes.
- Evaluate images before finalizing acquisition.
- If you get lost, go back to a known structure (e.g. LV at 0°).
- Comfortable positioning for the echocardiographer helps to obtain the best images possible.

2.3.3 TOE 2D scanplanes

DTG – Deep Transgastric

		DTG view
		45 – 50 cm
		Advance deep into stomach and anteflex
		0°
	2D	AV, Ao-root evaluation
	CFD	AV
	Doppler	AV (AS, AR)

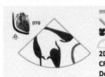

		DTG RV-inflow view
		45 – 50 cm
		Advance deep into stomach and anteflex
		100-130°
	2D	AV, Ao-root evaluation
	CFD	AV
	Doppler	AV (AS, AR)

TG – Transgastric

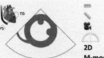

		TG Mid-SAX view
		40 – 45 cm
		Advance probe and anteflex slightly, withdraw from DTG
		0°
	2D	Mid-LV myocardium (function, thickness), pericardium, RV turn right
	M-mode	Dimensions (FS), area (FAC), myocardial thickness
		Biplane to TG 2-chamber view

		TG IVC LAX view
		40 – 45 cm
		Advance probe and anteflex slightly and turn
		right, withdraw from DTG
		30°
	2D	Liver, hepatic veins, IVC and RA (partial)
	M-mode	Dimension and respiratory variation IVC
	Doppler	Hepatic vein flow

		TG two chamber view (TG 2C view)
		40 – 45 cm
		Start from TG Mid SAX, anteflex slightly, withdraw for MV
		90°
	2D	LV myocardium (inferior and anterior), papillary muscles, chordae, MV
	M-mode	Dimensions (FS), myocardial thickness
		Biplane to TG mid SAX

		TG LAX view
		40 – 45 cm
		Start from TG Mid SAX, anteflex slightly
		120°
	2D	LVOT, AV
	CFD	LVOT, AV
	Doppler	LVOT, AV

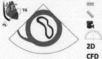

		TG basal SAX
		40 cm
		Withdraw from TG Mid SAX, anteflex slightly
		0°
	2D	Basal LV myocardium, MV ('fish mouth')
	CFD	MV

ME – Mid-Oesophageal

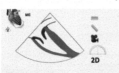

ME Coronary sinus view
40 cm
Withdraw from TG basal SAX or advance from ME four chamber view
0°
2D Coronary sinus for retrograde cardioplegia canulla or CRT-wire

ME four chamber view
35 - 40 cm
Withdraw from TG Mid SAX, retroflex
0°
2D LV function (septal and lateral walls), RV, MV, TV, pericardium
3D LV, MV, RV, TV
CFD TV, MV
M-mode TAPSE, MAPSE
Doppler Transmitral flow, transtricuspid flow, Tissue Doppler
⚹ Biplane to ME two chamber

ME AV SAX
35 - 40 cm
30°- 40°
2D AV, Coronary arteries
CFD AV, Coronary arteries

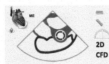

ME RV in - outflow
35 - 40 cm
60°
2D TV, TV, PV, RVOT, proximal PA
CFD TV, PV, RVOT

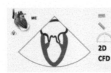

ME bicommissural view
35 - 40 cm
60°
2D MV (P3,A2,P1), (LAA)
CFD MV

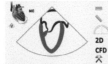

ME two chamber view
35 - 40 cm
90°
2D LV function (inferior and anterior walls), MV, (LAA)
CFD MV
⚹ Biplane to ME four chamber

		ME LAX view (TG LAX)
		35 – 40 cm
		120°
	2D	LV (Anteroseptal and inferolateral walls),LVOT, AV, MV (P2,A2),LA
	CFD	MV, LVOT, AV
	Doppler	MV, LVOT

		ME AV LAX view (TG AV LAX)
		35 – 40 cm
		Zoom from ME LAX
		120°
	2D	MV, AV, Ao root (dimensions)
	CFD	MV, LVOT, AV
	Doppler	MV, LVOT

		ME bicaval view
		35 - 40 cm
		110 – 120°
	2D	RA, IAS, SVC, <ivc
	CFD	IAS. (PFO, ASD...)

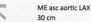

		ME asc aortic SAX
		30 cm
		120°
	2D	SVC, Ao, PA
	CFD	PA
	Doppler	PA

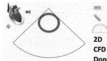

		ME asc aortic LAX
		30 cm
		90°
	2D	Ao
	CFD	Ao
	Doppler	Ao flow reversal

		desc Ao SAX
		35 - 40 cm
		0°
	2D	Ao
	CFD	Ao
	Doppler	Ao flow reversal

		desc Ao LAX
		35 - 40 cm
		90°
	2D	Ao
	CFD	Ao
	Doppler	Ao flow reversal

UE – Upper-Oesophageal

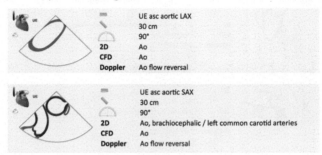

	▬	UE asc aortic LAX
	╲	30 cm
	◠	90°
	2D	Ao
	CFD	Ao
	Doppler	Ao flow reversal

	▬	UE asc aortic SAX
	╲	30 cm
	◠	90°
	2D	Ao, brachiocephalic / left common carotid arteries
	CFD	Ao
	Doppler	Ao flow reversal

2.3.4 TOE 3D views

Three-dimensional (3D) images are an integral part of an examination. However, 3D requires optimal 2D image quality, and the cost of 3D is (mainly) temporal resolution. Use ECG-gating when possible and minimize the window (x,y,z).

3D can be used as:
- Live mode (thick slice for visualizing structures and foreign objects).
- Zoom (valves, e.g., measurements left ventricular outflow tract (LVOT) area).
- Colour flow Doppler (CF Doppler) (visualize jets → increase wall filters).
- Full volume (LV and right ventricular (RV) volumes and LV strain/strain rate).

Workflow

1/ Optimize the 2D image.
2/ Then adjust gain, brightness and smoothing.
3/ Crop/rotate to display the 3D image according to guidelines or preferences.

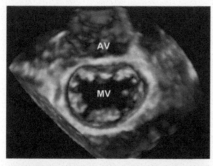

3D Zoom Mitral Valve Surgical view

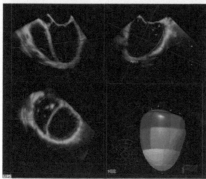

3D Full Volume of Left Ventricle

A number of **software-based analyses** may be performed. Following acquisition of 3D-datasets, vendor-specific built-in software can be used to perform offline measurements including LV function, mitral and aortic valve assessment. Also, vendor-specific speckle-tracking based strain and strain rate analyses exist for 2D and 3D. Similarly, dedicated software tools can be applied for the analysis of speckle-tracking based displacement, valve analyses, and RV analyses.

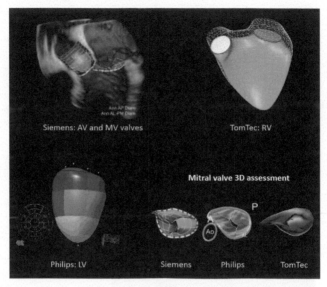

Siemens: AV and MV valves

TomTec: RV

Mitral valve 3D assessment

Philips: LV   Siemens   Philips   TomTec

2.4 References

1. Hahn RT, et al. *Guidelines for Performing a Comprehensive Transesophageal Echocardiographic Examination: Recommendations From the American Society of Echocardiography and the Society of Cardiovascular Anesthesiologists.* J Am Soc Echocardiogr. (2013) 26(9):921-64.
2. Kasper J, et al. *Additional Cross-Sectional Transesophageal Echocardiography Views Improve Perioperative Right Heart Assessment.* Anesthesiology. (2012) 117(4):726-34.

3

Left Ventricle: Systolic Function

JOHAN BENCE
STEFAAN BOUCHEZ

3.1 Anatomy

- Shape = a prolate ellipsoïd: elongated
  ellipse with a conical apex.
  - The shape has a major (base to
    apex) and a minor axis perpendicu-
    lar to the major axis with a ratio of
    2:1 in a normal LV.
  - Transversal circular shape: the inter-
    ventricular septum (IVS) between
    the LV and the RV functions as part
    of the LV, maintaining a circular
    shape during the cardiac cycle.

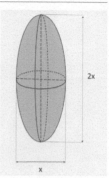

- Wall thickness (WT) of LV >> RV.
- 2 papillary muscles (PM): the posteromedial and the anterolateral PM.
- The apex of the heart is formed by the LV.
- Segmentation of the LV in correlation with the coronary artery
  anatomy accurately describes regional wall motion abnormalities (RWMA).

3.2 Physiology

- LV is a pressure chamber that pumps the oxygenated blood into
  the systemic circulation. The filling and ejection of blood is gen-
  erated by the helical arrangement of different myocardial layers.
- The systolic contraction relies on 3 movements:
  - The longitudinal shortening from base to apex.
  - The radial thickening inwards.
  - The circumferential torsion of the base clockwise and the
    apex counterclockwise.
- The LV is less compliant and less afterload dependent than the
  RV.

3.3 Echocardiography

3.3.1 Measurements of wall thickness and LV size

LV wall thickness
2D measurement of WT at end-diastole (ED) < 11 mm.
- TG Mid SAX view.
  - Inferolateral WT, excluding the PM.
  - Septal WT (in center of septum).

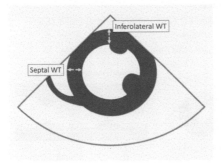

LV dimensions
Normal internal LV diameter measured at ED < 55mm or
< 32mm/m².

LV (DYS)FUNCTION	NORMAL	MILD	MODERATE	SEVERE
mm/m²	< 32	32-35	35-37	> 37
mm/ 1,75 m²	< 55	55 – 60	60 – 65	> 65

3.3.2 Global LV systolic function

- Assessment of LV systolic function is considered the foundation of echocardiography.
- LV performance can be assessed qualitatively (eye-balling, radial thickening) or quantitatively (measurements).

Fractional Shortening (FS)
- Based on linear measurements in the TG Mid SAX or TG LAX view.
- Measurement by M-mode:
  - LV internal diameters: ED (LVIDd) and end-systolic (ES) diameter (LVIDs).
  - Below the mitral valve (MV) leaflets and above the PM.

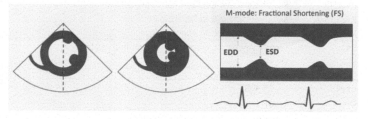

M-mode: Fractional Shortening (FS)

- Formula: FS % = $\dfrac{\text{LVIDd} - \text{LVIDs}}{\text{LVIDd}} \times 100$

LV (DYS)FUNCTION	NORMAL	MILD	MODERATE	SEVERE
FS %	> 25	25 – 21	20 - 16	<16

- Estimation of the ejection fraction (EF) from FS (Teichholz formula) is no longer recommended for clinical use.

Fractional Area Change (FAC)

- Based on areas in the TG Mid SAX view.
- Measured by tracing the LV endocardial border at ED (LV end-diastolic area: LV EDA) and ES (LV end-systolic area: LV ESA).

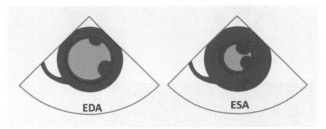

EDA   ESA

- Formula: $FAC \% = \dfrac{LV\ EDA - LV\ ESA}{LV\ EDA} \times 100$

LV (DYS)FUNCTION	NORMAL	MILD	MODERATE	SEVERE
FAC %	> 40	40 - 30	29 - 20	< 20

LV Ejection fraction

- LV-EF calculation is based on volumes and represents the percent of LV diastolic volume ejected during systole.
- Recommended method in 2D is the **Simpson's method of discs**.
  - Measurement by tracing the endocardial border of the LV at ED and ES. The LV length through the apex is indicated.
  - The software automatically determines the LV-EF and LV volumes: ED and ES.

LV (DYS)FUNCTION	NORMAL	MILD	MODERATE	SEVERE
2D LV-EF	> 55 %	54 - 45	44 -30	< 30

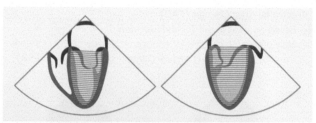

2D LV-EF: Simpson's method. Measurements in ME 4C and 2C at ED and ES

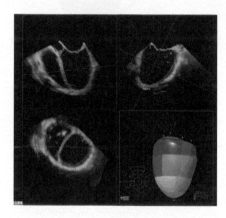

3D-based estimation of LV volumes and LV-EF

LV Ejection Fraction using 3D-TOE

- Global LV volumes and EF can be determined using a (semi-) automated border detection software.
- Measurement: Full Volume acquisition from the ME 4C view.

LV (DYS)FUNCTION	NORMAL	MILD	MODERATE	SEVERE
3D EDV ml / m²	< 75	75 - 85	86 - 96	> 97
3D ESV ml / m²	< 30	30 - 35	35 - 45	> 45
3D EDV ml / 1,75 m²	< 130	130 -150	150 -170	> 170
3D ESV ml / 1,75 m²	< 55	55 – 60	60 – 80	> 80

Mitral Annular Plane Systolic Excursion (MAPSE)

- Based on the longitudinal motion of the LV and is like TAPSE for the RV.
- Measured by M-mode in the ME 4C view, placing the examination beam on the lateral MV annulus.

LV (DYS)FUNCTION	NORMAL	MILD	MODERATE	SEVERE
MAPSE mm	> 11	10- 9	8 - 6	< 6

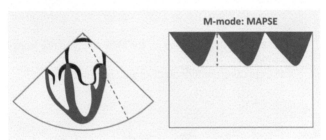

MAPSE

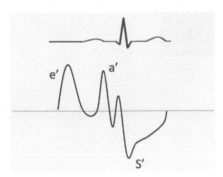

TDI lateral MV annulus

- MAPSE can also be assessed using the lateral MV Annular velocity S' by tissue Doppler imaging (TDI) in the ME 4C view. Normal LV S'$_{lat}$ > 8 cm/s (declines with age).

Systolic index of contractility dP/dt
- Assessment of LV global function.
- Measurement of dP/dt.
- During the isovolumic contraction period (before the AV opens when there is no significant left atrial pressure (LAP) change).
- Only useful for patients with more than mild mitral regurgitation (MR).
- Method:
  - Continuous Wave Doppler (CW Doppler) through MR in ME 4C view.
  - Measures the time required for the MR velocity to rise from 1 to 3 m/sec.
  - Calculate using the formula dP/dt = 32 mmHg/t.

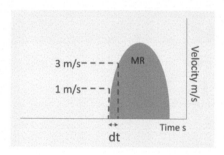

LV (DYS)FUNCTION	NORMAL	MILD	MODERATE	SEVERE
Time in msec (1-3 m/s)	< 27	27 - 40	40 - 64	> 64
mmHg/s	> 1200	1200 - 800	800 - 500	< 500

Global longitudinal peak systolic strain (GLPSS)

GLPSS analyzes myocardial deformation to assess LV systolic function. During the cardiac cycle the myocardium deforms in three dimensions:

- Longitudinal: shortening in the long axis of the myocardium.
- Circumferential: circumferential shortening or torsion of the myocardium.
- Radial: thickening of the myocardium.

Strain (ES-strain) describes:
- The deformation between two points within the myocardial wall.
- A % change from the initial length.
- A single dimensionless % parameter of deformation.

Methods to assess strain:
- TDI and 2D (3D) speckle tracking.
- Angle dependence is a limitation in TDI but not in speckle tracking.

$$\text{Formula Strain } (e) = \frac{L - L_0}{L}$$

- Negative strain during systole (fibers shortening): longitudinal and circumferential.
- Positive strain during systole (fibers thickening): radial.
- Method:
    - 2D acquisition (with high frame rate) of
        - ME 4C view.
        - ME 2C view.
        - ME LAX view.

- Application of speckle tracking software will display peak ES-strain as well as the average value for the global LV. When regional tracking is suboptimal in more than 2 myocardial segments in a single view, the calculation of GLPSS should be avoided.

Interpretation of GLPSS
- Normal LV systolic function.
  - **Longitudinal: <-20 % (GLPSS).**

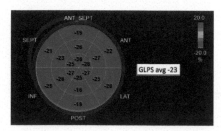

- LV dysfunction.
  - a relative reduction in GLPSS of > 15 % from baseline.
    (e.g. a decrease from – 21% to 17% identifies LV dysfunction)

3.3.3 LV regional function

LV segmentation to describe regional wall motion more accurately.
RWMA are correlated to a specific coronary artery region and
are described in a 17-segment LV model with the apex as the 17th
segment.
- Left anterior descending artery (LAD) : the anterior wall and
  2/3 of the IVS.
- Circumflex artery (Cx art.): the lateral wall.
- Right coronary artery (RCA): the RV and the inferior wall.

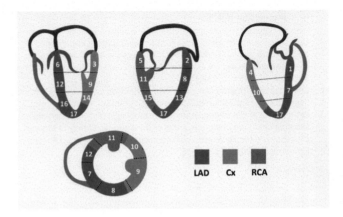

3.3.4 Summary

Systematic approach for the evaluation of LV systolic function.

1. LV dimensions and WT.
2. Global LV systolic function.
3. Ventricular septum: position.
4. Check MV: annular dilatation and MR.
5. Diastolic function: estimation of LV filling pressures.

3.4 References

1. Lang RM, et al. *Recommendations for Cardiac Chamber Quantification by Echocardiography in Adults: An Update from the American Society of Echocardiography and the European Association of Cardiovascular Imaging.* Eur Heart J (2015) 16: 233-271
2. Chengode S. *Left ventricular global systolic function assessment by echocardiography.* Ann Card Anaesth (2016) 19 (S1): 26-34
3. Reeves ST, et al. *Basic Perioperative Transesophageal Echocardiography Examination: A Consensus Statement of the American Society of Echocardiography and the Society of Cardiovascular Anesthesiologists.* J Am Soc Echocardiogr (2013) 26: 443-56.

4

Left Ventricle: Diastolic Function

STEFAAN BOUCHEZ

4.1   Introduction

- The guidelines for the evaluation of the diastolic function of the LV are not necessarily applicable for the intraoperative period.
- The dynamic changes in loading conditions (preload, after-load, heart rate…) make the utility of these echocardiographic diastolic parameters limited. Changes in diastolic parameters during the intraoperative period are due to changes in loading conditions and rarely due to changes in diastolic function.
- Definition:
  - = inefficient LV relaxation and compliance in diastole, impeding LV filling.
  - = an echocardiographic diagnosis.
- Diastolic heart failure:
  - = LV diastolic dysfunction and clinical signs of heart failure.
  - Aetiology of heart failure in 50% of patients.
- Phases during diastole.
  1/ Isovolumic relaxation phase: metabolic active process, start-ing after AV closure during which the LV pressure falls below the LAP opening the MV.
  2/ **Early filling** or rapid filling during further relaxation and 'suction' of LV.
  3/ Diastasis: as LV pressure equals LAP, flow across the MV drops.
  4/ **Atrial contraction**: the atrial contraction completes LV preload at ED. Contributes to 20% of LV preload in normal LV and up to 40% in diastolic dysfunction.

4.2   Echocardiography

4.2.1   Spectral Doppler

Mitral inflow

- Pulsed Wave Doppler (PW Doppler) at the MV leaflet tips in the ME 4C view.
- Measurements: the early filling (E), the deceleration time (DT) which is the slope from peak E to the baseline and the late atrial contraction (A).
    - Normal and pseudonormal pattern: E ≥ A   E/A >1
    - Impaired relaxation pattern: E < A   E/A <1
    - Restrictive pattern: E >> A   E/A >2
- Early filling E.
    - Early or rapid filling phase of LV filling.
    - Dependent on diastolic function and preload (increases with increased filling pressure) of the LV.
    - Is combined with TDI é to estimate LV filling pressure.
- Pulmonary vein flow (using PW Doppler):
    - Measured 1 cm in a pulmonary vein.
    - Early forward systolic flow, early forward diastolic flow and a late backward diastolic flow during atrial contraction.
        ◦ Normal: systolic dominance over diastolic flow.
        ◦ Diastolic dysfunction: a blunted systolic flow is found in marked diastolic dysfunction.
    - No longer recommended for the evaluation of diastolic function
- Colour M-mode transmitral flow Vp (Mitral Propagation Velocity).
    - Measures velocity of first column (E) of blood from left atrium (LA) to LV in the ME 4C view using CF Doppler. The cursor is placed parallel to the mitral inflow jet to measure the slope of early filling from the MV up to 4 cm into the LV cavity.
    - Vp has a weak evidence of correlation with filling pressures.
    - Normal Vp > 45 cm/sec.
      Abnormal Vp < 45 cm/sec.

4.2.2 Tissue Doppler Imaging

- TDI displays the myocardial velocities during systole and diastole. Usually measured at the lateral (or septal) myocardium at the level of the MV in the ME 4C view.
- TDI pattern has a
  - Systolic component S'.
  - Biphasic diastolic component: é and a'.
- TDI é.
  - A strong predictor of outcome.
  - Dependent on diastolic function and preload (decreases with increased filling pressure).
  - Is usually > 10 cm/s. A lower velocity indicates an impairment in LV relaxation.
  - The ratio E/é is a good estimate of LAP.
    - E/é > 14 indicates elevated LAP.
    - Formula by Nagueh: LAP = 1,24 x (E/é + 1,9)
    - Simplified formula: LAP = E/é + 4

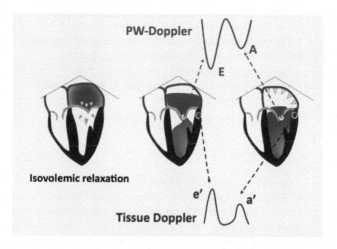

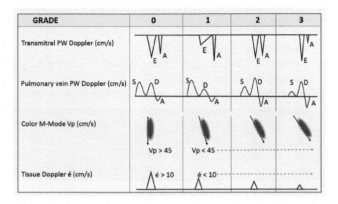

DIASTOLIC FUNCTION	NORMAL	GRADE 1	GRADE 2	GRADE 3
LV relaxation	normal	impaired	impaired	impaired
LAP	normal	normal/decreased	increased	increased
MV E/A m/s	1	< 1	> 1 < 2	> 2
E/é	< 10	< 10	10-14	> 14

- Simplified algorythm for the assessment of diastolic function.

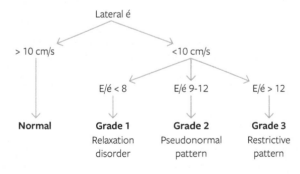

4.2.3 Summary: a 3-step approach for the evaluation of LV diastolic function

1/ Global systolic function: LV-EF.
2/ Estimate LV filling pressure: E/é and estimation of LAP + monitoring during surgery.
3/ Impairment of diastolic function: preload vs afterload sensitivity.

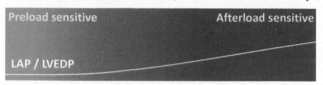

4.3 References

1. Swaminathan N, et al. *Utility of a simple algorithm to grade diastolic dysfunction and predict outcome after coronary artery bypass graft surgery.* Ann Thorac Surg (2011) 91: 1844-1850
2. Nagueh SF, et al. *ASE/EACVI Recommendations for the evaluation of left ventricular diastolic function by echocardiography.* J Am Soc Echocardiogr (2016) 29: 277-314

5

Right Ventricular Function

AN SCHRIJVERS
STEFFEN REX

5.1 Anatomy

- The RV is V-shaped with three parts:
  (1) Inlet including the tricuspid valve (TV), chordae tendineae, and PM.
  (2) Trabeculated apical myocardium.
  (3) Outlet including the infundibulum or conus and the pulmonic valve (PV).
- 3 PM (anterior, inferior, and medial or septal).
- Moderator band.
  - Bridging the RV cavity between the septum and parietal wall.
  - Protection from RV overdistension.
  - Perfused by LAD.
- Normally, the RV is not part of the apex of the heart.

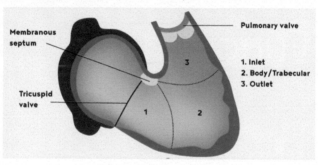

5.2 Physiology

- The RV is a
  - highly compliant (large increase in volume → minimal change in diastolic pressure),
  - afterload-dependent,
  - low-pressure pump.

- The RV supports LV preload and keeps the right atrial pressure (RAP) low.
- The RV has a peristaltic contraction pattern with sequential contraction of inflow-apex-outflow, simultaneous contraction in pressure overload. The RV ejection is a complex process with primarily a longitudinal contraction (systolic descent of the base) next to a circumferential contraction (free wall bellow effect). Due to ventricular interdependence, RV dysfunction/failure is inevitably associated with LV impairment/failure.
- RV failure is significantly correlated with a high mortality (up to 70%).

5.3   Echocardiography

5.3.1   Measurements of RV wall thickness and size

RV WT
- Normal RV WT measures < 5 mm at ED.
- Measurement:
  - TG SAX: inferior wall of RV.
  - ME 4C view: lateral wall of RV.

RV dimensions
The relative size of the RV should be compared with that of the LV: if the RV appears significantly larger than the LV, the RV should be reported as dilated despite measuring dimensions within the normal range.

	NORMAL (MEAN)	UPPER LIMIT	DILATATION
RV base cm	3,1 - 3,5	< 4,2	≥ 4,2
RV mid cm	2,3 - 3,3	≤ 3,5	> 3,5
RV length cm	6,7 - 7,5	≤ 8,3	> 8,3

ME 4C view measurments at ED

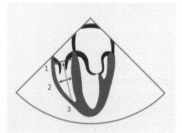

ME 4C RV dimensions at ED:
RV base (1), RV mid (2), RV length (dotted line 3)

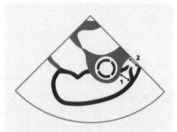

ME RV in-outflow RV outflow tract (RVOT) diame-
ters at ED RVOT (1),
Pulmonary artery (PA) (2)

		REFERENCE RANGE	MILDLY ABNORMAL	MODERATELY ABNORMAL	SEVERELY ABNORMAL
RVOT (PV)(1)	cm	1,7 - 2,3	2,4 - 2,7	2,8 - 3,1	≥ 3,2
PA diameter (PA)(2)	cm	1,5 - 2,1	2,2 - 2,5	2,6 - 2,9	≥ 3,2

- The basal diameter is defined as the maximal SAX dimension in the basal one third of the RV (ME 4C view).
- The mid cavity diameter is measured halfway between the basal diameter and the RV apex at the level of the PM.
- RV Length is measured from the TV annular plane to the RV apex.
- In all echocardiographic reports, the RV basal diameter should be reported.

Simplified 'indexed' values to define RVOT and PA diameter based on reference values and 1,75 m² BSA:

- RVOT at level of PV: > 24 mm (14 mm/m² indexed).
- PA diameter: > 21 mm (12 mm/m² indexed).

Ratio RV/LV area

- RV to LV size measured in ME 4C view by tracing the area.

RV DILATION	VENTRICULAR SIZE	APEX
Mild	Enlarged, RV EDA < LV EDA (usually < 0.7)	Apex includes LV
Moderate	RV EDA = LV EDA	Apex includes both RV and LV
Severe	RV EDA > LV EDA	RV extends beyond the LV

Ecccentricity index
- Eccentricity index (EI) using the TG mid SAX view:
  - D-shaping of the IVS.
  - Normal: EI = 1 at ED and ES.
    - RV volume overload (ED) EI > 1.
    - RV pressure overload (ES) EI > 1.

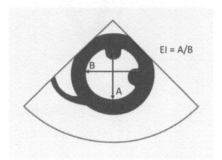

5.3.2　RV systolic function

RV performance can be assessed qualitatively (eye-balling, longitudinal shortening) or quantitatively (measurements).

Right Ventricular Ejection Fraction (RV-EF)
- Formula: RV-EF = [(RV EDV–RV ESV)/RVEDV] x 100 (%)
  EDV end-diastolic volume; ESV end-systolic volume.
- Normal RV-EF 44-71% vs abnormal < 44%.
  - 2D assessment is not recommended because of the numerous geometric assumptions.
  - 3D models of the RV better estimate RV volumes and EF.

RV Fractional Area Change (FAC)
- Formula: RV FAC = [(RV EDA - RV ESA) / RV EDA * 100 (%)

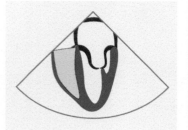

RV-EDA

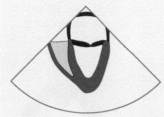

RV-ESA

	VIEW	NORMAL	IMPAIRED
RVFAC %	ME 4C	+/- 50	< 35

Tricuspid Annular Plane Systolic Excursion (TAPSE)
- TAPSE can be measured using
  - Anatomical M-mode (AMM) in the ME 4C view.
  - By assessing the annular-to-apical distance (AAD, in ME 4C) in diastole and systole. TAPSE = $AAD_D - AAD_S$.
  - Note that RV longitudinal motion is affected by pericardiotomy.

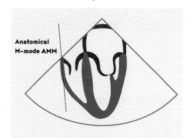

ME 4C view using anatomical M-mode AMM

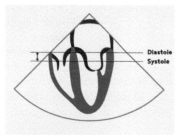

ME 4C view measuring annular to apical distance

	VIEW	NORMAL	IMPAIRED
TAPSE	ME 4C (AMM)	> 24 mm	< 16-17 mm
	ME 4C AAD	> 20-25 mm	
	TG RV inflow (AMM)		
	DTG RV inflow-outflow (AMM)		

Rate of rise of intraventricular pressure (dP/dt)
- Tricuspid regurgitation (TR) jet using CW Doppler.
- Measure the time (dt) between velocity (v) of 0.5 m/s and 2 m/s.
  - dP = according to the modified Bernoulli equation 15 mmHg.
  - dP/dt = 15 mmHg/dt.

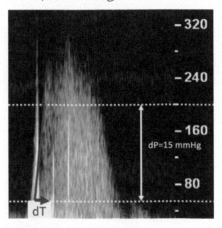

	NORMAL	IMPAIRED
dP/dt	> 400 mmHg/s	< 400 mmHg/s
	dt ≤ 37,5ms	dt > 37,5ms

Tricuspid Annulus Velocity (S')

TDI sample volume at the lateral annulus in TG or ME RV in-out view.

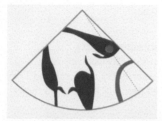

TG RV in-outflow

ME RV in-outflow

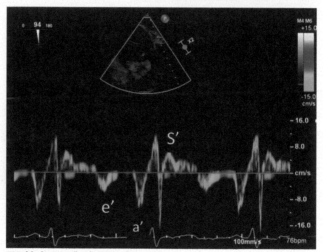

TDI of the free RV wall at the TV annulus

TDI	NORMAL	IMPAIRED
S' cm/s	> 9,8 – 16,4	< 9,5

Strain

- Speckle tracking software required.
- Strain = a percentage change in myocardial deformation (negative value).
- Estimates global and regional RV function.
- Global longitudinal peak systolic strain (GLPSS):
  - RV free wall strain: average strain of 3 RV-free wall segments (basal/mid +/- apical).
  - Global RV strain: average strain of 6 RV segments including free wall and septum (ME 4C view).

	NORMAL	IMPAIRED
RV free wall GLS	< - 27	> - 20
RV global GLS	< - 22	> - 16
	NORMAL	IMPAIRED
RV free wall GLS	< - 27	> - 20
RV global GLS	< - 22	> - 16

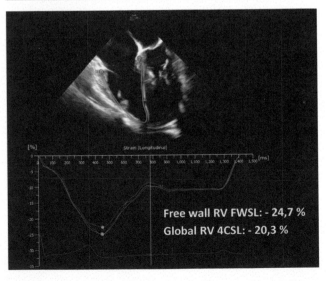

Free wall RV FWSL: - 24,7 %

Global RV 4CSL: - 20,3 %

5.3.3 RV diastolic parameters

Right ventricular filling pressures
IVC assessment
- Good correlation between right atrial pressure (RAP), IVC size and collapsibility index(relative decrease in IVC diameter with inspiration) in non-ventilated patients.
- The maximum and minimum diameters of the IVC with respiration/ventilation should be measured > 2 cm from the RA.
- Spontaneously breathing patients:
  - IVC collapsibility index:
    - CI = (IVC max-IVC min)/IVC max (%)
    - maximum diameter at end-expiration, minimum diameter at end-inspiration.
- Mechanically ventilated patients:
  - IVC distensibility index:
    - DI = (IVC max-IVC min)/IVC min (%)
    - maximum diameter at end-inspiration, minimum diameter at end-expiration.

	RAP 3 MMHG (0 – 5 MMHG)	RAP 8 MMHG (5-10 MMHG)	RAP 15MMHG (10 -20 MMHG)
IVC diameter	< 2,1 cm	2,1	> 2,1 cm
Collapsibility Index	> 50%	no manifest variation	< 50%

TV Doppler
- PW Doppler at the TV leaflet tips in the ME 4C view.
  - Measurements: the early filling (E) and the late atrial contraction (A).
  - as the TV is larger than the MV, the inflow velocities are lower.
- Tissue Doppler Imaging (TDI).
  - Measurement of TV annular motion: é.

- Estimation of filling pressure: ratio E/é.
  - Normal: E/e' < 6.
  - Elevated RAP: E/e' > 10.
  - Limited reference data, accurate measurements are difficult (angle dependency!).

Hepatic venous flow using PW Doppler

IMPAIRED RELAXATION	PSEUDONORMAL	RESTRICTIVE
S/D >1 Adur > 50% S	S/D < 1	S reversed
RAP 5 mmHg	RAP 10-15 mmHg	RAP > 15 mmHg

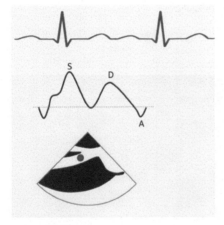

Hepatic vein Doppler tracing

Pulmonary artery pressure assessment
Systolic pulmonary artery pressure (sPAP)
- Assessment of systolic pulmonary artery pressure (sPAP) using CW Doppler.
- Used to diagnose pulmonary arterial hypertension (PAH).
- Method:
  - CF Doppler to detect the presence of TR.
  - TR jet velocity: CW Doppler in ME RV inflow-outflow view or ME modified bicaval view.
    - RVSP − RAP = 4 $(TR)^2$
    - sPAP = RVSP (in the absence of pulmonic stenosis (PS))
    - sPAP = 4 $(TR)^2$ + RAP

	NORMAL	SEVERE PAH
TR velocity m/s	< 2,5	> 3,5
sPAP mmHg	< 30	> 50

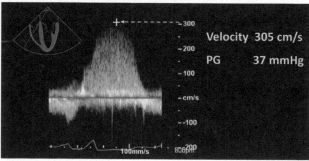

Velocity 305 cm/s

PG 37 mmHg

TR jet velocity using CW Doppler

Pulmonary artery acceleration time (PACT)

- Used to diagnose PAH.
- PW Doppler at the level of the PV.
  - Time interval from the beginning of RV ejection to peak flow velocity across the PV.
  - Estimation of mean pulmonary artery pressure (mPAP): PAT 100 msec correlates with mPAP 25mmHg or using the formula: mPAP = 79 – 0,45(PACT).

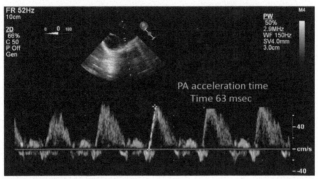

PACT measurement using PW Doppler.

SEVERITY	PACT MSEC
Normal PAP	> 120
Borderline PAH	100-120
PAH	< 100

RV volume and pressure overload
- ME 4C and TG mid SAX.

McConnell's sign
- Sign of acute regional RV dysfunction.
- Preserved contraction of the RV apex with akinesis of the free wall.
- Sign of acute RV pressure overload.

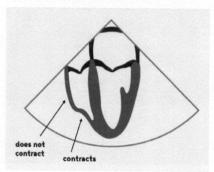

does not contract   contracts

McConnell's sign

Chronic Volume Overload
- RV dilatation.
- Paradoxical septal motion in <u>diastole;</u> D-shaping of the LV.
  - In severe primary TR and PR.
  - In left-to-right shunts at the atrial level.

Chronic Pressure Overload

- RV dilatation.
- RV hypertrophy (ME 4C at ED).
- Paradoxical septal motion in <u>systole</u>; D-shaping of the LV.
  - PS.
  - Severely elevated pulmonary vascular resistance (PVR).

	Enddiastole	Endsystole
Normal		
Volume overload		
Pressure overload		

Eccentricity index changes in pressure- and volume overload.

5.3.5 Summary: systematic approach for the evaluation of RV function

1. RV dimension and WT.
2. Global RV systolic function.
3. IVS: position.
4. Check TV: annular dilatation and TR.
5. Determine RV filling pressures: RAP, PAP.

5.4   References

1. Haddad F, et al. *The right ventricle in cardiac surgery, a perioperative perspective: anatomy, physiology, and assessment*. Anesth Analg (2009) 108(2):407–21.
2. Vegas A. (2018). *Perioperative two-dimensional transesophageal echocardiography*. A practical handbook. (2nd ed.) Springer International Publishing AG.
3. Rudski LG, et al. *Guidelines for the Echocardiographic Assessment of the Right Heart in Adults: A Report from the American Society of Echocardiography*. J Am Soc Echocardiogr (2010) 23:685-713.

6

Aortic Valve

STEFAAN BOUCHEZ

6.1 Anatomy

The AV and the aortic root.

- Aortic outflow tract: AV, aortic root and ascending aorta.
- Aortic root: ventriculo-arterial junction (VAJ) → three sinuses of Valsalva (SVS) ← sinotubular junction (STJ). There is no true ring-shaped AV annulus, instead a virtual ring formed by the basal cusp attachments at the VAJ.
- Aortic valve: 3 cusps.

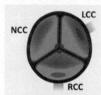

  - Left coronary cusp (LCC): ostium left coronary artery.
  - Right coronary cusp (RCC): ostium right coronary artery.
  - Non-coronary cusp (NCC): no ostium.
- Normal AV area in adults: 3 – 4 cm^2.
- Bicuspid valve (BAV):
  - 2 types (Sievers Classification).

    ∘ Type 0: symmetrical cusps of same size, no raphe.
    ∘ Type 1: most common is a BAV with 2 functional cusps of unequal size with a raphe in the largest cusp.

Type 0

  - Associations:
    ∘ Aortic stenosis (AS) at young age and aortic regurgitation (AR).
    ∘ Root or ascending aorta dilatation.
    ∘ Aortic coarctation.
    ∘ Patent ductus arteriosus.
    ∘ Ventricular septum defect (VSD).
    ∘ Anomalous coronary implantation.

Type 1

6.2 Physiology

The AV is a complex structure that allows a unidirectional flow of blood out of the LV, optimizes of the coronary blood flow, and supports the preservation of myocardial function. Its shape allows for distribution of the exposed stresses such that the AV will function without complications throughout a lifetime.

6.3 Echocardiography

- Annulus or VAJ:
  inner-to-inner edge in mid-systole.
  - 3D preferred over 2D, since the VAJ is not circular and dynamic during cardiac cycle.
- SVS, STJ and Asc Aorta:
  leading to leading edge at ED.
- Aortic WT < 2 mm.

NORMAL SIZE (MM) ME LAX	VAJ - ANNULUS	SVS	STJ	ASC AO
Diameter / 1,75 m²	27	37	30	32
Diameter / m²	< 15	< 21	< 17	< 18

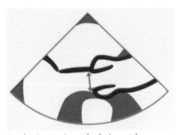

Annulus: inner-to-inner edge during systole

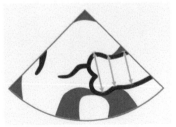

Aorta: leading to leading edge during diastole

6.4 References

1. Loukas M, et al. *The anatomy of the aortic root.* Clin Anat. (2014) 27(5):748-56.
2. Hahn RT, et al. *Guidelines for Performing a Comprehensive Transesophageal Echocardiographic Examination: Recommendations from the American Society of Echocardiography and the Society of Cardiovascular Anesthesiologists.* J Am Soc Echocardiogr (2013) 26:921-64

7

Aortic Regurgitation (AR)

MICHEL VAN DYCK
MARIA ROSAL MARTINS
GUILLAUME LEMAIRE

7.1 Definition

Aortic regurgitation (AR) is the diastolic backflow of blood from the aorta into the LV leading to volume overload of the LV, a widened pulse pressure and a decrease in cardiac output.

7.2 Aetiology

VALVE LEAFLETS	AORTIC ROOT
Congenital: bicuspid, unicuspid. Degenerative disease: leaflet prolapse Endocarditis: leaflet perforation Rheumatic valve disease Traumatic injury of the leaflets	Connective tissue disease: Marfan Aortic dissection Aortitis, etc.

7.3 Functional classification

AR Classification	Type 1				Type 2 Cusp prolapse	Type 3 Cusp restriction
	Ia	Ib	Ic	Id		
Mechanism						
Primary repair	STJ repair Asc. Ao. graft	AV sparing surgery	Subcommissural annuloplasty (SCA)	Patch repair	Prolapse repair	Leaflet repair

7.4 Echocardiography

7.4.1 2D/3D assessment

AV
- Cusp number: tricuspid – bicuspid – (unicuspid/quadricuspid).
- Cusp mobility: calcification and cusp thickness.
- Closure /coaptation defect: prolapse, dilatation, perforation.
- Commissural orientation (especially in BAV).
- Coronary implantation (especially in BAV).
- Coexisting laesions: vegetations, tumors, abscesses, etc.

Aortic root
- Dilatation of SVS, STJ and/or aorta.
- Dissection of aorta.
- Differentiation of syndromes: associated pathology.

LV
- Severe AR in presence of normal LV size indicates the presence of acute AR.
- LV size gradually increases with chronic AR.
- Asymptomatic AR: consider surgery in a dilated LV:
  - LV end-systolic diameter (LV-ESD): 20 >< 25mm/m^2.

Colour flow Doppler
- Nyquist velocity at 50-60 cm/sec.
- Jet direction:
  - Central jet: usually annular dilatation.
  - Eccentric jet: cusp prolapse, BAV, restricted leaflet.
  - Jet length into LV correlates poorly with AR severity.
- Jet diameter versus LVOT diameter measured in ME LAX and 1 cm from the AV is commonly used to grade AR.

- **Vena Contracta** (VC) is the smallest diameter of the jet at the level of the AV. The values of multiple jets cannot be added. VC area can also be measured using 3D-multiplanar reconstruction (MPR).
  - Method:
    - Best measured in ME AV LAX.
    - Optimize colour gain/scale (50-60 cm/s).
    - Identify the three components of the jet (VC, PISA, jet into LV), zoom and measure the smallest VC.
    - A VC > 6 mm is consistent with severe AR.

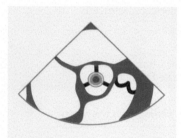

AR in ME AV SAX

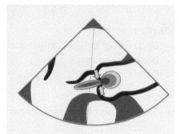

AR in ME AV LAX
Vena Contracta width (yellow arrows)

Spectral Doppler

- **Pressure half-time (PHT)**: CW Doppler is used to measure AR flow in the DTG or TG LAX view. The rate of decline of the AR jet velocity can quantify the AR by measuring the PHT. If the pressure between the aorta and the LV equilibrates fast, a severe AR must be present.
- **Aortic flow reversal** in the descending aorta is measured with PW Doppler. Holodiastolic flow reversal in the distal aorta is associated with severe AR. The ratio of flow reversal to forward flow (Velocity Time Integral (VTI)-ratio) can also serve as an indicator for AR severity.

8

Aortic Stenosis

MAHESH PRABHU

8.1 Definition

Aortic stenosis (AS) represents obstruction of blood flow across the aortic valve due to pathologic narrowing. The increased pressure gradient between the LV and the aorta leads to LV hypertrophy, diastolic dysfunction and in a later stage systolic dysfunction.

8.2 Aetiology

Supravalvular	Membrane
Valvular	Senile calcification
	Congenital BAV
	Rheumatic disease
Subvalvular	Membrane
	HOCM/SAM

8.3 Echocardiography

8.3.1 2D/3D assessment

- AV
  - Number of leaflets: tricuspid – bicuspid –(unicuspid/quadricuspid).
  - Cusp mobility and separation: calcification and cusp thickening.
  - Commissural fusion and orientation (especially in BAV).
  - Closure /coaptation defect: associated AR.
  - Coronary implantation (especially in BAV).
- Aortic root.
  - Poststenotic dilatation.
- LV.
  - LV hypertrophy (LVH).
  - Regional Wall Motion Abnormalities (RWMA): 30% coronary artery disease involvement.

Colour flow Doppler
- Nyquist velocity at 50-60 cm/sec.
- AV: quick screening tool to detect the level of obstruction by turbulent flow: valvular or not. Also identifies the presence of AR.
- MV: functional MR often present due to high systolic pressures.

Spectral Doppler
- Velocities.
  - Measurements in the DTG or TG LAX view.
    ◦ across AV using CW Doppler.
    ◦ In the LVOT using PW Doppler.
  - AV velocity.
    ◦ Normal AV or mild AS: triangular (early peaking) contour. Normal velocity over AV should be < 1 m/s.
    ◦ Severe AS: parabolic shape.
    ◦ LVOT obstruction: dagger-shaped contour (late peaking).
- **_Dimensionless Velocity Index (DVI)_ _or_ _Velocity Ratio:_**
  - CW Doppler measurement reveals a double envelop pattern in AS.
    ◦ The LVOT low-velocity contour is the inner 'brighter' envelop.
    ◦ The high velocity AS contour is the outer less dense envelop.
    ◦ PW Doppler can be used to measure LVOT velocity if the LVOT velocity is difficult to visualize in the double envelop.
    ◦ DVI compares the maximum velocity in the LVOT to the maximum velocity through the AV. AS is present when the AS velocity is 4 times higher than the LVOT velocity or when the DVI < 0,25.

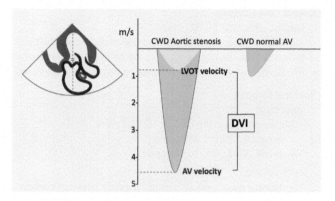

- Pressure gradient (PG) over the AV.
  - PG is the difference between the LV pressure and the concomitant pressure in the aorta.
  - The peak instantaneous PG is calculated using the Bernouilli equation:
    - Simplified: $\Delta P = 4 \times V^2_{max}$ if $V_{LVOT} < 1$ m/s
    - Modified: $\Delta P = 4 \times V^2_{max} - V^2_{LVOT}$ if $V_{LVOT} > 1,5$ m/s
  - The mean gradient is obtained by tracing the CW Doppler contour or can be estimated using $\Delta P_{mean} = 2,4 \times V^2_{max}$
- Catheterization versus echo-Doppler:
  - Measurement of valvular gradient.
  - Doppler measures instantaneous gradient.
  - Catheterization measures peak to peak gradient.
  - Mean gradient between Doppler and catheterization will be very similar.

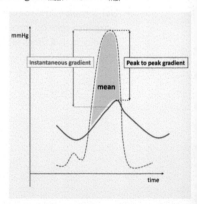

- Pressure recovery.
  - Source of discrepancy between catheterization and echo-Doppler. The aortic pressure measured by catheterization distal to the orifice is higher than at the orifice (Pressure recovery). The gradient measured by CW Doppler measures the highest velocity at the level of the orifice and does not take the pressure recovery into account.
  - The kinetic energy of blood accelerated though the stenotic orifice is partially recovered as pressure downstream in the aorta. In most cases pressure recovery has a negligible effect on the accuracy of the gradient calculation but is more prominent in small, non-dilated aortas (<30 mm).

Aortic Valve Area (AVA)
- **Planimetry:** estimation of the smallest anatomic AV orifice in the ME AV SAX.
  - Acoustic shadowing caused by the heavy calcifications often cause difficulties in measuring the orifice area.
  - 3D-MPR may help to locate the smallest orifice at maximal leaflet separation.
  - The average area of a non-stenotic three-cusped AV, can be measured by measuring the length of a cusp (L) and applying the following formula: $AVA = 0{,}433 \times L^2$

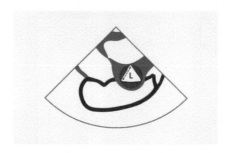

- **Continuity equation**: this applies the conservation of mass principle which states that blood flow or stroke volume (SV) over different valves is equal.

  Formula: $SV_{LVOT} = SV_{AV}$

  $CSA_{LVOT} \times VTI_{LVOT} = CSA_{AV} \times VTI_{AV}$

  $CSA_{AV} = \dfrac{CSA_{LVOT} \times VTI_{LVOT}}{VTI_{AV}}$

  $CSA_{LVOT} = \pi \times r^2$ or $\pi \times \dfrac{(D_{LVOT})^2}{2^2}$ or $0{,}785 \times D_{LVOT}^2$

  CSA: Cross Sectional Area in cm^2.

  D_{LVOT} = diameter LVOT measured in ME LAX from inner-to-inner edge.

  3D-MPR helps to localize the D_{LVOT} as this is not circular and often a source of error.

  Simplified equation: use of velocities instead of VTI.

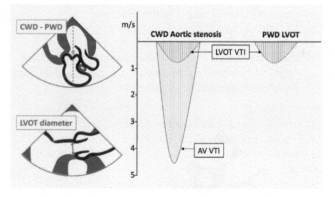

AORTIC STENOSIS	NORMAL	MILD	MODERATE	SEVERE
Peak jet velocity m/s	1,4 – 2,2	2,2 – 2,9	3,0 – 4,0	>4,0
Peak gradient mmHg	<20	20 – 40	40 – 70	>70
Mean gradient mmHg	-	<20	20> <50	>50
DVI or Velocity ratio	-	>0,50	0,50 – 0,25	<0,25
AVA cm²	3 – 4	1,5	1,5 – 1	<1
AVA cm² / m²		>0,85	0,85 – 0,60	<0,60
LV Hypertrophy	-	-	+	++

8.3.3   Summary: assessment of AS

1. Number of leaflets.
2. Amount of calcification of annulus and leaflets.
3. Annular size.
4. Presence and severity of AR.
5. Peak and Mean AV gradient.
6. LV function + degree of LVH and septal hypertrophy.

8.4   Concurrent echocardiographic conditions

8.4.1   LV Hypertrophy

- Caused by valve obstruction results in a small ventricular cavity, thick walls and diastolic dysfunction. Remember that the presence of increased WT may also suggest hypertrophic cardiomyopathy or an infiltrative disease like amyloidosis.
- Small SV may cause lower velocity and PG.

8.4.2 Low-flow, low-gradient AS

- **with poor LV-EF.**
- LV systolic dysfunction + severe AS.
- Effective Orifice Area (EOA) <1.0 cm^2, LV-EF < 40% and mean gradient < 40 mmHg.
- Consider dobutamine to increase CO:
  - Mean gradient increases with the increase in CO: true AS.
  - AVA increases with the increase in CO: pseudo-AS.
- **with preserved LV-EF**
  - Elderly patients with hypertension, hypertrophied, small volume LV, reduced longitudinal LV function and fibrosis.
  - EOA <1.0 cm^2, LV-EF < 40% and mean gradient < 40 mmHg, Stroke Volume index (SVi) SVi < 35 mL/m^2 and high calcium load.

8.4.3 Co-existing AR

- Trans-aortic volume flow rate, maximum velocity, and mean gradient increases with severe co-existing AR and is higher than expected for a given valve area.

8.4.4 Co-existing MR

- MR may be caused due to LV pressure overload.
- With severe MR, a low trans-aortic flow will cause a low AS gradient.
- Conversely a high LV pressure due to AS may overestimate jet size of MR.

8.4.5   Co-existing Mitral Stenosis (MS)

- MS contributes to low flow, low gradient AS.

8.4.6   Co-morbidities

- High CO states (anaemia, arteriovenous fistula) may cause relatively high gradients in the presence of mild or moderate AS.
- Aortic root dilation, associated with BAV disease, should be measured using the ME AV LAX view and the impact of pressure recovery should be noted.
- Hypertension may affect flow and gradients but not AVA.

8.5 References

1. Baumgartner H, et al. *Recommendations on the echocardiographic assessment of aortic valve stenosis: a focused update from the European Association of Cardiovascular Imaging and the American Society of Echocardiography.* Eur Heart J Cardiovasc Imaging. (2017) 18(3):254-275.
2. Baumgartner H, et al. *Echocardiographic assessment of valve stenosis: EAE/ASE recommendations for clinical practice.* J Am Soc Echocardiogr. (2009) 22(1):1-23.
3. Nishimura RA, et al. *2014 AHA/ACC Guideline for the Management of Patients with Valvular Heart Disease: executive summary: a report of the American College of Cardiology/American Heart Association Task Force on Practice Guidelines.* Circulation. (2014) 10;129 (23):2440-92.

9

Aorta

ANGELA MAHDI
STEFAAN BOUCHEZ

9.1 Anatomy

Tubular structure, divided into five segments:

- **Aortic root:** from the aortic valve (AV) to the sinotubular junction (STJ).
  - Contains:
    - AV annulus.
    - AV cusps.
    - Two coronary ostia.
    - Three sinuses of Valsalva (SVS).
- **Tubular ascending aorta**: from the STJ to the brachiocephalic artery.
- **Aortic arch**: from the brachiocephalic artery to the left subclavian artery.
- **Descending thoracic aorta**: from left subclavian artery to diaphragm.
- **Abdominal aorta**: from the diaphragm to the bifurcation.

The aortic wall is composed of three layers.

- Tunica intima (interna).
- Tunica media.
- Tunica adventitia (externa).

TOE cannot distinguish these layers when aortic wall is normal. Diseases such as dissection and atheroma alter aortic wall anatomy.

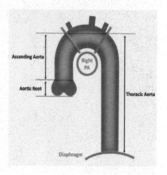

9.2   Physiology

The aorta is the most proximal artery connected directly to the heart. It acts both as a conduit and an elastic chamber. In its latter role, the aorta's elasticity serves to convert the heart's pulsatile flow to nearly steady flow in peripheral vessels.

The aortic diameter varies with age, sex, body size
- Rate of aortic expansion: 0.9 mm in men vs 0.7 mm in women for each decade of life.
- Upper normal limit of aortic diameters: 40 mm.

9.3   Echocardiography in pathology

9.3.1   Thoracic aortic aneurysm

Definition
An aneurysm is a permanent, localized arterial dilation to more than 50% of the normal diameter.
- Aortic dilatation between 3,7 and 5 cm.
- Aneurysm > 5 cm.

Anatomy
- Aortic dilatation which contains all three layers of the aortic wall.
  - Saccular or fusiform shape.
- Size: > 1.5 x normal diameter.
- Location:
  - Ascending aorta in 50% of cases.
  - Descending aorta in 40% of cases.
  - Aortic arch in 10% of cases.
- Associated findings: AR, thrombus, atheroma.

Aetiology

Leaflets	Congenital: Ebstein
	Inflammatory/Infectious: Rheumatic/Endocarditis
	Trauma: Blunt/Pacemaker leads
	Other: Myxomatous/Carcinoïd
Annulus	Idiopathic: Atrial fibrillation
	Secondary to RV dysfunction/dilatation
Ventricle	RV overload: Shunts
	RV myopathy: Myocardial infarction, Cardiomyopathy
	Increased pulmonary vascular resistance: Cor pulmonale, LV disease

Crawford classification

I   Below left subcalvian artery to above renal arteries.
II Below left subclavian artery to the bifurcation.
III 6th intercostal space to bifurcation.
IV 12th intercostal space to bifurcation.
V   6th intercostal space to above renal arteries.

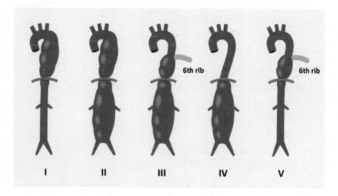

Indications for surgery
- > 55 mm.
- > 50 mm:
  - BAV + risk factors*.
  - Marfan without risk factors*.
- > 45 mm:
  - Marfan + risk factors*.
  - AV surgery.

*Risk factors: Age, atherosclerosis, hypertension, smoking and family history.

Echocardiography
Measurements
- From *leading edge to leading edge* at ED.
- Exception: AV annulus from *inner edge to inner edge* in mid systole.

Pre-CPB
- Location,shape and extent of the aneurysm.
  - Dilation.
  - Increased echogenicity of aortic wall.
  - Spontaneous contrast 'smoke'.
- Dimensions in ME LAX.
  - AV annulus, SVS, STJ and the ascending aorta (at the level of right PA).

Dimension in ME Ao SAX – LAX.
  - Descending aorta.
- Presence of haematoma or mural thrombus.
- Assessment of the AV:
  - Dilation of AV annulus.
  - AR.
    - Severity.
    - Mechanism.
- Assessment of biventricular function.

Post- CPB
- Evaluation of the graft and proximal anastomosis.
- Assessment of AV competence: presence of AR.
- Biventricular function.

9.3.2 SOVA: Sinus of Valsalva Aneurysm

Definition

Congenital or acquired dilatation of a SVS which may usually rupture in right heart chambers.

Anatomy

SOVA arises from:
- – Right SVS in 70% of cases.
- – Non SVS in 25% of cases.
- – Rarely from the left SVS.

- Associations:
  - – VSD in about 50% of cases.
  - – AR in 25% of cases.

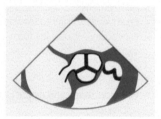

Ruptured non SVS aneurysm into right atrium

Echocardiography
- 2D/3D.
  - – Fingerlike 'windsock' image.
  - – CF Doppler for the direction of from SVS to chamber.

9.3.3 Aortic dissection

Definition

A disruption between the intima and the media of the aortic wall, creates a dissection of the two layers creating a false and a true lumen.

Aetiology

- Dilated aorta (aneurysm).
- Expectant (pregnancy).
- BAV.
- Aortopathy (atherosclerosis and connective tissue disease).
- Coarctatio aortae.
- Iatrogenic (trauma, surgery).

Debakey and Stanford classification

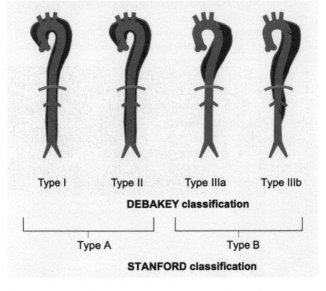

Indication for surgery

- Type A is a surgical emergency.
- Type B: surgical management in presence of complications:
  - Impending rupture.
  - Poor visceral or limb perfusion.
  - In connective tissue disease.

Echocardiography (Type A)

Pre-CPB

- Confirmation of the diagnosis.
    - Presence of an intimal flap: mobile structure within the vessel.
    - Presence of a true and false lumen.

- Artefacts.
    - Reverberation artefacts: atherosclerotic wall, PA catheter.
    - Sidelobe artefacts from the AV.

- Location of the dissection and entry site (disruption of the intimal flap usually > 5mm).
    - Assessment with 2D/3D, M-mode and CF Doppler.
    - In 70% of cases within the first few cm above the SVS.
    - In 25% of cases at the ligamentum arteriosum.
    - In some cases, no exact localization.
        ∘ In case of multiple tears.
        ∘ Location at blind spot of aortic arch.

- Coronary artery involvement.
    - In about 15% of cases.
    - Flap in relation to coronary arteries should be evaluated.
    - RWMA.
    - CF Doppler to assess ostial coronary blood flow.

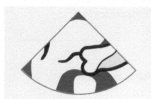

ME LAX: *dissection flap in asc Ao.*
White = true lumen.

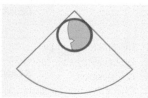

ME desc. Ao: *dissection flap and entrance tear.*
White = true lumen.

- False versus true lumen.

	TRUE LUMEN	FALSE LUMEN
Lumen	Smaller	Larger
Expansion	Systolic	Diastolic
Echogenicity inner layer	Poor	Bright
Low flow / thrombus	Absent	Present
Colour flow Doppler	Prominent systolic	Variable

- Aortic regurgitation.
  - In about 60% of cases.
  - Mechanism:
    ○ Dilatation of aortic root.
    ○ Destruction of AV annular support with cusp prolapse.
    ○ Disturbance of cusp closure by presence of haematoma at the annulus.
    ○ Dissection flap prolapse into AV.
- LV function.
  - Global LV function.
  - Increased WT due to hypertrophy is often present (due to chronic hypertension).
  - RWMA: coronary artery involvement causing myocardial ischemia.
- Pericardial and pleural effusion.
  - Rupture or leak of the dissection.
  - Risk of tamponade.
  - Transudation is more common than blood by rupture.

Post-CPB
- False lumen: absence of flow indicates successful closure of the communication.
- Biventricular function.
- AR: AV competency after repair of the dissection.

9.3.4 Aortic intramural haematoma

Definition

A localized separation of the aortic wall layers without the presence of an intimal flap or dissection tear.

Echocardiography
Criteria.

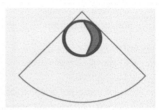

- No intimal flap.
- Aortic WT $\geq$ 7 mm.
- Extent 1 – 20 cm.
- A layered appearance.
- Absence of flow.

9.3.5 Penetrating atherosclerotic ulcer

Definition

An atherosclerotic laesion with ulceration causing a thickened aortic wall. (descending >> ascending aorta).
Progressive penetration may result in

- Intramural haematoma.
- Aneurysm.
- Dissection.

Echocardiography
Ulcer appears as a calcified focal outpouching or 'crater' of the aortic wall +/-.

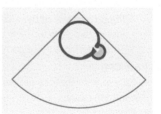

- Aneurysm.
- Intramural haematoma.
- Dissection of the concomitant aneurysm.

9.3.6 Aortic atherosclerosis

Definition

Atherosclerosis causes thickening of the intima of the aortic wall with luminal irregularities.

Echocardiography

- Irregular thickening of the intimal aortic wall.
- Plaques:
  - Appear brighter: tissue density and presence of calcium.
  - Possible artefacts: acoustic shadowing.
  - Need for accurate description of laesions.
    - Location.
    - Thickness.
    - Mobile structures.

9.3.7 Classification or grading (Adapted from Katz)

GRADE	DESCRIPTION	INCIDENCE OF STROKE %	IMAGE
1	Normal aorta	0	
2	Extensive thickening < 3 mm	0	
3	Protruding < 5 mm into aortic lumen	5	
4	Protruding > 5 mm into aortic lumen	10	
5	Mobile atheromata of any size	50	

9.4   References

1. Hiratzka LF, et al. *ACCF/AHA/AATS/ACR/ASA/SCA/SCAI/SIR/STS/SVM Guidelines for the diagnosis and management of patients with thoracic aortic disease. A Report of the American College of Cardiology Foundation/ American Heart Association Task Force on Practice Guidelines, American Association for Thoracic Surgery, American College of Radiology, American Stroke Association, Society of Cardiovascular Anesthesiologists, Society for Cardiovascular Angiography and Interventions, Society of Interventional Radiology, Society of Thoracic Surgeons, and Society for Vascular Medicine.* Circulation (2010) 121: 266-369
2. Evangilista A, et al. *Echocardiography in aortic diseases: EAE recommendations for clinical practice.* Eur J. Echocard. (2010) 11: 645-658
3. Evangelista A, et al. *The current role of echocardiography in acute aortic syndrome.* Echo Res Pract (2019) 6: 53-63

10

The Mitral Valve

STEFAAN BOUCHEZ

10.1 Anatomy

The MV apparatus is an anatomical term describing all cardiac structures associated with MV function and includes the annulus, the leaflets, the chordae, PM and the LV.

- The annulus is saddle shaped.
  - Lowest points at the commissures.
  - Highest points at the middle of the anterior-posterior annulus.
  - Shape changes during cardiac cycle: large circular diastolic shape versus smaller systolic D-shape.
  - MV annulus area 4-6 cm². Surface area is twice the annulus area which allows for large coaptation area (30%).

- The MV leaflets: anterior (AMVL) and posterior (PMVL) leaflet.
  - Leaflet thickness < 4 mm.
  - AMVL.
    - Largest semicircular leaflet.
    - Covers 30 % of the annular circumference.

  - PMVL.
    - Smaller leaflet, approximately half the size of the AMVL.
    - Covers 70 % of the annular circumference.
    - 3 incomplete identations, creating 3 scallops.

  - Carpentier's nomenclature (see figure).

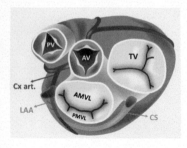
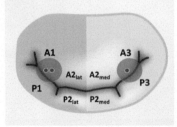

- Chordae tendineae.
  - Fibrous chords or strings connect the MV leaflets to the PM and the LV wall.
    - Anterior PM attach to A1, lateral A2, P1 and lateral P2.
    - Posterior PM attach to A3, medial A2, P3 and medial P2.
  - Three orders of chordae:
    - 1st order: free margins of the leaflets, preventing prolapse.
    - 2nd order: body of leaflet, reducing tension.
    - 3nd order: LV wall to base of PMVL.
- Papillary muscles.
  - 2 PM: anterior (anterolateral) and posterior (posteromedial).
    - Anterior PM has dual blood supply: Cx art. and LAD.
    - Posterior PM has single vessel blood supply: Cx art. or RCA.
      - More vulnerable for ischemia and rupture (VSD).

10.2 Physiology

The normal MV is a dynamic structure that permits blood to flow from the LA to LV during diastole and sealing of the LA from the LV during systole. The MV apparatus prevents backflow of blood and pressure from the LV to the LA and the pulmonary circulation. Pathology of the MV apparatus may lead to pulmonary oedema and pulmonary hypertension.

10.3 Mitral Regurgitation

Definition
MR is caused by the retrograde flow of blood from the LV into the LA through the MV, leading to volume overload of the LV and pressure overload of the pulmonary circulation.

Aetiology
- Myxomatous degeneration: Fibroelastic degeneration, Barlow disease.
- Congenital: endocardial cushion defect or associated with other pathologies.
- Endocarditis.
- Cardiomyopathy: dilated (including ischemic), restrictive, hypertrophic.
- Rheumatic: often accompanied by MS.
- Inflammatory: systemic lupus, rheumatoïd arthritis.

Functional classification by Carpentier

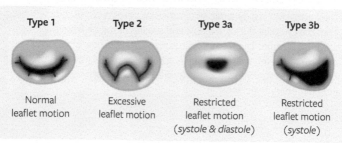

Type 1	Type 2	Type 3a	Type 3b
Normal leaflet motion	Excessive leaflet motion	Restricted leaflet motion (*systole & diastole*)	Restricted leaflet motion (*systole*)

2D-TOE assessment.
- MV annulus.
  - MV annular dilatation:
    - Diastolic ratio annulus/anterior leaflet in ME LAX is > 1.3
    - MV annular diameter is > 35 mm.
  - Calcification (MAC) and extent.
- Leaflets.
  - Detailed description of:
    - The precise location of the involved leaflets/ scallops.
    - The description of the presence and extent of calcifications and/or vegetations.
    - The extent of anatomic changes.
  - Leaflet thickening (>5 mm), malcoaptation (including pro-lapse and flail), vegetations and calcifications.
  - Leaflet lengths: measurement of leaflet lengths.
    - AMVL: 12 – 14 mm/m^2.
    - PMVL: 5 – 8,5 mm/m^2. A length > 15 mm is a risk factor for SAM after MV repair.
- Left atrium:
  - Progressive increases in MR leads to LA dilatation. LA dilatation and the loss of sinus rhythm also play a role in MV dysfunction.
  - Presence of spontaneous echo contrast or 'smoke'.
  - Clots may be present, especially in the left atrial appendage (LAA) (thrombi < 2 mm can be missed).
  - TOE LA diameter is best measured in ME AV SAX or ME LAX. LA size is usually underestimated by TOE compared with TTE.
  - LA size:
    - < 40mm: normal
    - > 50 mm: severe dilatation and often present in MR.
    - > 60 mm: cryoablation is not recommended.

3D-TOE assessment.

- Advantages:
  - Improves the visualization and accuracy of interpretations of MV pathology.
  - The ability to visualize the entire MV apparatus in real time and the image can be manipulated to reveal structures from angles not available in 2D.
- En-face or surgical view.
  - Routinely generated using the 3D zoom mode based on the ME 4C view. The size and position of the two zoom boxes of X-plane images are adjusted and optimized to include the whole MV. The acquired 3D image can then be rotated to display the MV en-face from the LA with the AV directly above it at the 12 o'clock position.
- The 3D datasets can be used for the offline 3D quantitative assessment of the MV using semi-automated analysis software which:
  - Generates a colour-coded parametric model of the MV.
  - Allows the depiction of the pathology in one single image.
  - Generates serial MV measurements, including MV annular size, leaflet coaptation length, tenting height, billowing volume and leaflet areas.

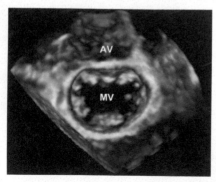

En face view of the MV

Colour flow Doppler (CF Doppler).

- MR jet area:
  - The jet area of the regurgitant jet is not recommended to quantify the severity of MR. The CF Doppler imaging should be used for detecting MR.
  - A jet area > 50% of LA area or a wall hugging jet are consistent with severe MR.

- Vena Contracta.
  - Refers to the narrowest part of the MR jet, just distal to the anatomical orifice and represents the regurgitant orifice.
  - Best measured in ME LAX view.
  - Optimize colour gain/scale (50-60 cm/s).
  - Identify the three components of the jet (VC, PISA, Jet into LA), zoom and measure the smallest VC.
  - A VC > 7 mm is consistent with severe MR.

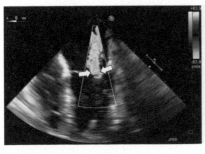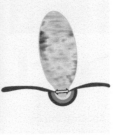

- Proximal isovelocity surface area (PISA).
  - Used to calculate effective regurgitant orifice area (EROA).
  - In MR, flow accelerates and converges as it approaches the regurgitant orifice. This flow convergence creates hemispheric shells of increasing velocities on the upstream side of the regurgitant orifice. The instantaneous flow at any of these shells is equal to the flow at the regurgitant orifice at the same moment (conservation of mass principle).

- PISA method:
  - Optimize CF Doppler imaging of MR.
  - Zoom the image of the MR regurgitation
  - Decrease the Nyquist limit: Baseline shift of CF Doppler in direction of flow to induce aliasing on the ventricular side of the MV.
  - Measure PISA radius by measuring the distance from first aliasing to the regurgitant orifice (=radius).
  - Simplified method: Set Nyquist at 40 cm/s and measure radius. A radius >9 mm is consistent with severe MR.
  - CW Doppler through the MR to measure the maximal MR velocity.

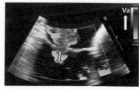
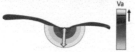

PISA flow = regurgitant orifice flow
  or
PISA x V_A = EROA x $V_{max.}$ (PISA = 2π r^2)
  or
$$EROA = \frac{(2\pi\ r^2 \times V_A)}{V_{max}}$$

Regurgitant volume ml = EROA x MR VTI cm

Spectral Doppler.
- PW Doppler of the MV and pulmonary veins.
  - Transmitral flow: When E-wave dominance and > 1,2 m/s, consider moderate to severe MR. A-wave dominance excludes severe MR.
  - Pulmonary vein flow: systolic flow reversal is highly specific for severe MR while a normal pattern (S>D) predicts none or mild MR.

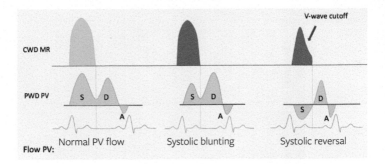

CWD MR

PWD PV

Flow PV: Normal PV flow   Systolic blunting   Systolic reversal

- CW Doppler of MR jet.
  - Density of waveform: consider severe MR when contour is dense and triangular shaped (early peaking).
- Continuity method.
  - When both MV and AV function are normal: $SV_{MV} = SV_{LVOT}$
    When MR is present: $SV_{MV} > SV_{LVOT}$
    $$SV_{MV} = (MVA \times VTI_{MV}) \text{ in ml}$$
    $$SV_{LVOT} = CSA_{LVOT} \times VTI_{LVOT} \text{ in ml}$$
    MR regurgitant volume = $SV_{MV} - SV_{LVOT}$ in ml.
  - The fraction of SV that regurgitates through an incompetent MV is called the regurgitant fraction (RF) in %.

Severity grading of MR.

MITRAL REGURGITATION		GRADE 1 MINIMAL MR	GRADE 2 MODERATE MR	GRADE 3	GRADE 4 SEVERE MR
Anatomy	Valve	Normal or abnormal	Normal / abnormal		Flail / PM rupture
	LV ESD mm/m²	< 22			> 22
CF Doppler	Jet area %	< 20	20 - 50		> 50
	2D VC mm	< 4	4 - 6		> 6
	3D VC area cm²	< 0,20	0,20 – 0,40		> 0,40
	PISA radius mm	< 4	4 - 9		> 9
PW Doppler	Mitral inflow	A dominance	variable		E dominance (> 1 , 4 m/s)
	PV flow	S ≥ D	S Blunting		S reversal
	VTI MV/VTI AV	< 1	1 – 1,4		> 1,4
CW Doppler	Density MR	Faint parabolic	Moderate parabolic		Dense – triangular
Calculation	EROA cm²	< 0,20	0,20 – 0,29	0,30 – 0,40	> 0,40
	RV ml	< 30	30 – 44	45 – 60	> 60
	RF %	< 30	30 - 50		> 50

Systolic Anterior Motion of Anterior MV leaflet or SAM.

Definition.
- Defined as a 'dynamic' displacement of the distal portion of the anterior leaflet of the MV toward the LVOT causing LVOT obstruction and MR.

Associations.
- Post MV repair.
- Hypertrophic cardiomyopathy.
- Hypertensive heart disease.

Physiologic conditions:
- Hyperadrenergic state (inotropic stimulation).
- Decreased preload.
- Decreased afterload.

Echocardiographic risk factors:
- Septal hypertrophy >15 mm in diastole.
- Anterior MVL > 20 mm in diastole.
- Posterior MVL > 15 mm in diastole.
- AL:PL $\leq$ 1,3 at onset systole.
- C-sept (coaptation-septum distance) $\leq$ 25 mm at onset systole.
- Mitro-aortic angle < 120° at onset systole.

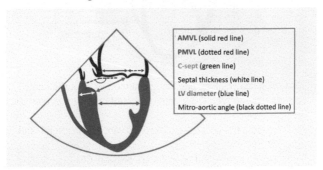

AMVL (solid red line)
PMVL (dotted red line)
C-sept (green line)
Septal thickness (white line)
LV diameter (blue line)
Mitro-aortic angle (black dotted line)

Secondary (functional) MR.

Definition.
Moderate to severe MR due to coronary artery disease (LV re-modeling after myocardial infarction) in the absence of primary or preexisting leaflet or chordal pathology. Most cases of functional MR fall into Carpentier type 3b (systolic restriction), although Carpentier type 1 (annular dilatation) often coexists.

Echocardiography.
When dealing with unfavourable echocardiographic characteristics, annuloplasty alone often fails in these patients.

Unfavourable characteristics:
- Tenting height > 10 mm.
- Tenting area > 2.5 cm².
- P3 scallop tenting angle > 29°.

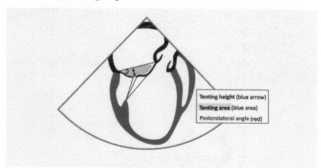

Tenting height (blue arrow)
Tenting area (blue area)
Posterolateral angle (red)

LV remodelling:
- Interpapillary muscle distance 20 mm.
- Posterior papillary-fibrosa distance > 40 mm.
- Lateral wall motion abnormality.
- LV EDD > 65 mm and/or LV ESD > 51 mm.
- Systolic sphericity index (Major / Minor axis) > 0.7 (Biplane sphericity index can be calculated as an average of the SAX and LAX length in the 4- and 2-chamber views).

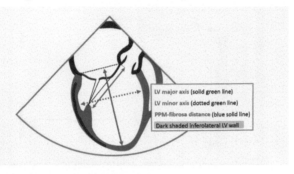

LV major axis (solid green line)
LV minor axis (dotted green line)
PPM-fibrosa distance (blue solid line)
Dark shaded inferolateral LV wall

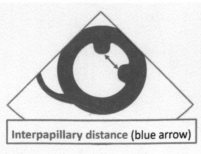

Interpapillary distance (blue arrow)

MR treatment decision tree.

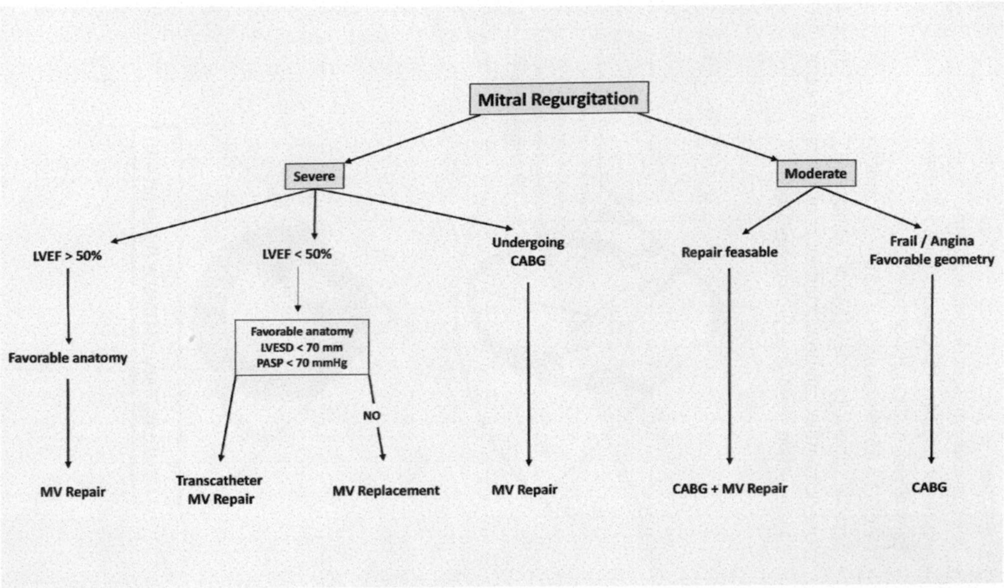

MV repair versus replacement.

Contraindications for repair: factors considered unsuitable for repair and favorable longterm results.

- Preexisting MS.
- Presence of severe MAC with a mean transmitral gradient > 3 mmHg.
- Infectious MV leaflet destruction.
- Emergency surgery with ischemic PM rupture.
- Severe ischemic MR with unfavorable MV and LV geometrical indices.

10.3.2 Summary: intraoperative assessment of MR.

1. Establish the presence of MR.
2. Quantify the MR.
3. Exclude contraindications for repair.
4. Identify the mechanism of MR: Carpentier's classification.
5. Identify the underlying pathophysiologic laesion: dilated annulus, posterior posterior leaflet flail, etc.
6. Assess and quantify the geometric indices in ischemic MR.
7. Exclude the presence of predictors of repair failure: SAM, etc.
8. Evaluation post repair/replacement.
   a. Localize and quantify any residual MR: valvular or paravalvular.
   b. Mean gradient over MV: MS secondary to MV repair.
   c. Global and regional LV function (Cx art.).
   d. Presence of SAM.
   e. AV: new AR due to capture of NCC with ring sutures.

10.4 Mitral stenosis

10.4.1 Definition

Mitral stenosis (MS) is a narrowing of the MV orifice, impeding forward diastolic flow of blood from the LA towards the LV. The pressure overload in the LA causes LA dilatation and leads to pulmonary hypertension which may impede RV function.

10.4.2 Aetiology

- Rheumatic valvular disease.
- Degenerative/calcific MS.
- Systemic lupus erythematosus.
- Congenital MS.
- Rheumatoid arthritis.

10.4.3 Echocardiography

2D/3D structural assessment of MV apparatus
- Mitral Annular Calcification (MAC).
- Cusps:
  - Mobility:
    - Rheumatic MS: diastolic doming of the AMVL with 'hockey stick' deformity.
    - MAC: restricted motion of PMVL.
    - Thickening: leaflet tips > 3mm.

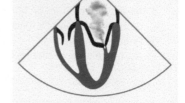

  - Calcification:
    - Rheumatic MS: 'frozen' anterior leaflet.
    - MAC: annular calcification among PMVL.

- Commissural and subvalvular fusion with chordal shortening in rheumatic MS.
- Left atrium:
  - Dilated (often atrial fibrillation).
  - Presence of spontaneous echo contrast or 'smoke'.
  - Clots may be present (LAA).
- Mitral Leaflet Separation Index (MLS index).
  - Semiquantitative method that measures the distance between the leaflet tips in ME 4C or ME LAX view.
  - Non severe < 1,2 cm vs severe < 0,8 cm.
- Planimetry.
  - 2D ME Basal SAX view: not recommended.
  - 3D MV: after 3D acquisition, MPR is used to identify the maximal opening of the MV leaflets through the cardiac cycle. Planimetry can be performed by tracing the smallest opening of the MV.

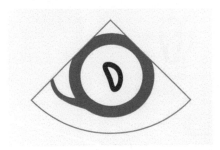

2D ME Basal SAX view (not recommended for planimetry)

Colour Flow Doppler
- **Proximal Isovelocity Surface Area (PISA):**
  - Mitral Valve Area (MVA) calculation by using the flow convergence zone in the left atrium (less validated method).
  - Combines CF Doppler to measure the radius of the aliasing hemisphere and the maximal velocity across the MV using CW- or PW Doppler.

- PISA is not affected by LV compliance.
- PISA can be useful in the presence of
  AR and/or MR.

$$MVA \times Vmax = 2\pi r^2 \times V_{alias}$$
$$MVA = 6.28 \, r^2 \times (V_{alias} / Vmax)$$
$$MVA \, (MS) = 6.28 \, r^2 \, (\alpha° / 180°) \times (V_{alias} / Vmax)$$

Spectral Doppler
Gradient across the MV.

- Mean PG is calculated by tracing the MV inflow and better
  estimates MS severity using CW Doppler in the ME 4C view.
  Visualization of flow direction using CF Doppler may help ensure
  adequate alignment.
- Mean PG:
  - overestimates MS in tachycardia and MR.
  - underestimates MS in low CO and AR.

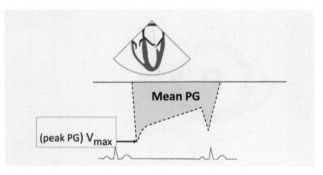

Pressure half-time (PHT).

- The rate of decline of a PG across the orifice is determined by the area.
- In case of bimodal slope, it is more accurate to trace the PHT-slope in mid-diastole, than tracing the early deceleration slope.
- PHT is the time in milliseconds for the peak PG to decrease in half: MVA = PHT/220
- PHT is related to DT: PHT = 0,29 x DT
  - Deceleration time is the time from peak pressure to zero: MVA= 759/DT
- PHT measurements rely on pressure differences and flow through the MV. Abnormal PHT measurements alter the MVA assessment.
  - Is shortened and underestimates MVA in AR, ASD, high CO and low LV compliance.
  - Is prolonged and overestimates MVA in low CO, hypovolemia.

Continuity method.

- Calculation of MVA by comparing flow across the MV with the flow over LVOT or AV. There should be no LVOT obstruction, AR or MR.
- Formula: $MVA= \dfrac{CSA_{LVOT} \times VTI_{LVOT}}{VTI_{MV}}$

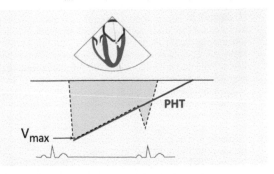

Severity grading of MS

MITRAL STENOSIS	NORMAL	MILD	MODERATE	SEVERE
Area cm^2	4 - 6	2,5 - 1,5	1,5 - 1,1	≤ 1
Mean PG mmHg	-	< 5	5 - 10	> 10
PHT ms	< 90	90 - 150	150 - 220	≥ 220

10.4.4 Summary: assessment of MS.

1. Mobility of leaflets and presence of sheet calcification of AMVL.
2. Fused commissures.
3. Subvalvular fusion / chordal shortening.
4. MAC.
5. MVA and PG over MV.
6. RV function and presence of pulmonary hypertension.

10.5 References

1. Mahmood F, et al. A practical approach to an intraoperative three-dimensional transesophageal echocardiography examination. J Cardiothor Vasc Anesth (2016) 30: 470 - 490
2. Sliwa K, et al. Rheumatic heart disease: the tip of the iceberg. Circulation (2012) 125: 3060 - 3062
3. Lancellotti P. et al. *Recommendations for the echocardiographic assessment of native valvular regurgitation: an executive summary from the European Association of Cardiovascular Imaging.* European Heart Journal – Cardiovascular Imaging (2013) 14, 611–644
4. Zoghbi WA. Et al. *Recommendations for Noninvasive Evaluation of Native Valvular Regurgitation: A Report from the American Society of Echocardiography Developed in Collaboration with the Society for Cardiovascular Magnetic Resonance.* J Am Soc Echocardiogr. (2017) 30(4):303-371.
5. Mahmood F. et al. *Echocardiographic Assessment of the Mitral Valve for Suitability of Repair: An Intraoperative Approach From a Mitral Center.* J Cardiothorac Vasc Anesth. (2022) 36(7):2164-2176.
6. Carpentier A, et al. Carpentier's Reconstructive Valve Surgery. 1st edition Saunders (2010) ISBN 978-0721691688

11

Tricuspid Valve

ISABELLE MICHAUX

11.1 Anatomy

- Largest cardiac valve: 8-12 cm^2 and has lowest transvalvular gradient.
- In a normal heart, the TV is located slightly closer to the apex than the MV.
- 3 leaflets: Anterior (largest) > Septal > Posterior.
  - Often more leaflets in 50% of patients: 4 leaflets (2 posterior leaflets).

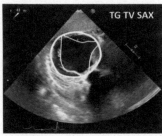

Tricuspid Valve: TG TV SAX with three leaflets.

- Papillary muscles
  - Anterior PM, attached to the moderator band.
  - Posterior PM sometimes absent.
  - Septal PM.
- Fibrous annulus
  - Triangular and saddle-shaped.
  - Little fibrous tissue, susceptible to dilatation.

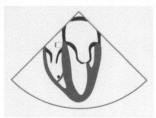

TV has a more apical position than MV: blue arrows; Moderator band*

11.2 Physiology

The right heart is coupled to the systemic venous return and the pulmonary circulation. The TV by preventing backward flow, supports the RV to keep venous pressures low and to push the blood towards into the pulmonary circulation. Pathology of the TV may lead to venous congestion and organ dysfunction.

11.3 Tricuspid regurgitation

11.3.1 Definition

TR is caused by the retrograde flow of blood from the RV into the RA through the TV, leading to volume overload of the RV and pressure overload of the systemic circulation.
- Physiologic TR (in 75% of normal individuals) is associated with normal TV anatomy and RV function.
- Pathological TR is usually secondary to a dilated TV Annulus (TA), RV dilatation and leaflet tethering (functional TR).

11.3.2 Aetiology

Leaflets	Congenital: Ebstein
	Inflammatory/Infectious: Rheumatic/Endocarditis
	Trauma: Blunt/Pacemaker leads
	Other: Myxomatous/Carcinoïd
Annulus	Idiopathic: Atrial fibrillation
	Secondary to RV dysfunction/dilatation
Ventricle	RV overload: Shunts
	RV myopathy: Myocardial infarction, Cardiomyopathy
	Increased pulmonary vascular resistance: Cor pulmonale, LV disease

11.4 Echocardiography

Tricuspid Annular (TA) dilatation
- TA measured at ED (peak QRS) in the ME 4C view.
- ED diameter of > 40-42 mm or > 21-23 mm/m².
- TA diameter in 2D underestimates the actual diameter measured by 3D (LAX view of TV).
- Good correlation between the TA diameter and the TR volume.
- 3D acquisition and 3D MPR:
  - 3D Zoom acquisition of TV.
  - 3D MPR to measure 3D LAX diameter.

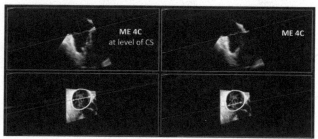

TV diameter (yellow arrow) at level of coronary sinus or in center of ME 4C view

Colour Flow Doppler

TR jet area
- The area of the regurgitant jet is not recommended to quantify the severity of TR. The CF Doppler should be used for detecting TR.
- A jet area > 50% of RA area or a wall hugging jet are consistent with severe TR.

Vena Contracta

- Refers to the narrowest part of the TR jet, just distal to the anatomical orifice and represents the regurgitant orifice.
- Best measured in ME 4C view.
- Optimize colour gain/scale (50-60 cm/s).
- Identify the three components of the jet (VC, PISA, Jet into RA), zoom and measure the smallest VC.

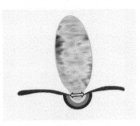

- A VC $\geq$ 7 mm is consistent with severe TR.
- Ratio VC/TA_{ED} > 0,24 is associated with poor prognosis in secondary TR. (TTE).
  - Proximal isovelocity surface area (PISA):
    - Used to calculate effective regurgitant orifice area (EROA).
    - Method: see chapter on MR.
    - A PISA > 9 mm indicates severe TR.

Spectral Doppler

PW Doppler of TV and hepatic veins

- Transtricuspid flow: When E-wave dominance and > 1 m/s, consider moderate to severe TR.
- Hepatic vein flow: systolic flow reversal suggests severe TR.
  - RA dilatation may eliminate this finding.
  - May be seen in atrial fibrillation and pacing.

CW Doppler of TR jet

- Density of waveform relative to antegrade flow.
- Peak TR jet velocity reflects instantaneous gradient across the TV. The pressure difference estimates RVSP and PAP in absence of RVOT obstruction.

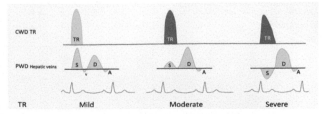

TRICUSPID REGURGITATION	MILD	MODERATE	SEVERE
STRUCTURAL MODIFICATIONS			
Leaflet coaptation	Body-to-body	Edge-to-edge	Absent
Leaflet thetering (mm)	None	<8	>8
Annular diameter (mm)	< 40	> 40	> 40
RV and RA size	Normal	Normal >< dilated	Dilated
IVC diameter (mm)	<20	21-25	>25
QUALITATIVE DOPPLER			
Colour Flow jet area	Small, narrow	Moderate central	Large central or eccentric jet
Flow convergence (PISA)	Absent or small	Intermediate in size and duration	Large, visible throughout the systole
CW Doppler density & contour	Soft, partial, parabolic	Dense, parabolic	Dense, triangular
SEMIQUANTITATIVE DOPPLER			
CF Doppler jet area (cm²)	Not defined	Not defined	>10
Vena contracta (cm)	< 0.3	0.3-0.69	≥ 0.7
PISA radius (cm)	≤ 0.5	0.6-0.9	> 0.9
Hepatic venous flow	Systolic dominance	Systolic blunting	Systolic reversal
Tricuspid inflow (m/sec)		Variable	E > 1.0
QUANTITATIVE DOPPLER			
EROA (cm²)	<0.2	0.2-0.39	≥ 0.4
Regurgitant vol (ml)	< 30	30-44	≥ 45

TR	MILD	MODERATE	SEVERE	MASSIVE	TORRENTIAL
Vena contracta cm	<0,30	0,30 - 0,69	0,70 - 1,30	1,40 - 2,00	≥ 2,10
EROA cm²	<0,20	0,20 - 0,39	0,40 - 0,59	0,60 - 0,79	≥ 0,80
3D Vena contracta Area cm²	-	-	0,75 - 0,94	0,95 - 1,14	≥ 1,15

11.5 Tricuspid stenosis

11.5.1 Definition

Tricuspid stenosis (TS) is a narrowing of the TV orifice, impeding forward diastolic flow of blood from the RA towards the RV. The pressure overload in the RA causes RA dilatation and leads to pulmonary hypertension which may impede RV function.

11.5.2 Aetiology

TS is relatively uncommon: rheumatoid, carcinoïd.

11.5.3 Echocardiography

Severity grading of TS

TRICUSPID STENOSIS	MILD	MODERATE	SEVERE
Leaflets and mobility	Normal	Thickened and moderately restrictive	Calcified, diastolic doming
Right atrial size	Normal	Dilated	Severely dilated
E peak velocity (cm/s)	< 0,7	> 0,7	> 1,5
PHT (msec)			> 190
Mean gradient (mmHg)	< 2	2-4	> 5

11.6 References

1. *Vahanian A, et al. 2021 ESC/EACTS Guidelines for the management of valvular heart disease.* Eur Heart J. (2022) 43(7): 561-632
2. Lancellotti P, et al. *Recommendations for the echocardiographic assessment of native valvular regurgitation: an executive summary from the European Association of Cardiovascular Imaging.* Eur Heart J - Cardiovascular Imaging (2013) 14 (7): 611–644.

12

Pulmonic Valve

JENS FASSL
JAKOB MATTHAEUS LABUS
CHRISTOPHER UHLIG

12.1 Anatomy

- Pulmonic valve (PV) is part of the pulmonary root complex connecting RVOT to PA.
- PV usually lies superior, anterior and left to the AV.
- Pulmonic root is cylindric shaped and consists of 3 components (PV, RVOT, PA).
- Pulmonic valve:
  - Semilunar 3 crescent-shaped valve.
  - Cusps named in relation to AV (right, left, anterior).
  - Size of the PV similar to AV, but cusps are typically thinner.
  - Normal PV Area is 2 – 4 cm^2.
  - Normal PV Annulus 28 ± 5 mm.

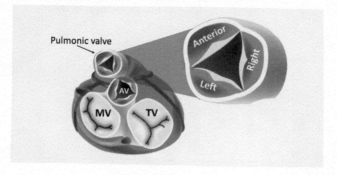

- Right Ventricular Outflow Tract (RVOT).
  - Cylindric RV infundibulum.
  - Independent of interventricular septum and TV.
  - No fibrous support of PV.
  - RV musculature in direct continuity with sinus of PA.
- Pulmonary Artery.
  - Dilates slightly forming sinuses of Valsalva.
  - PA annulus not well-defined (evaluation at the level of cusps insertion).

12.2 Physiology

The PV separates the RV from the PA and prevents the back flow of blood from the PA to the RV.

12.3 Pulmonic regurgitation

Mild ('physiologic') pulmonic regurgitation (PR) can be found in up to 80% of patients, moderate and severe PR is rare.

Primary PR	Congenital	Morphologic PV anomalies (bicuspid or quadricuspid PV, PV hypoplasia), post-repair of Tetralogy of Fallot, PV prolapse
	Acquired	Infective endocarditis, rheumatic, carcinoid, trauma
Secondary PR (functional)	Dilated PA or RVOT (volume-related due to left-to-right shunts)	
	Pulmonary embolism	
	PAH (acute or chronic)	

12.4 Echocardiography

12.4.1 2D/3D TOE

Annulus dilatation
- dilatated PA or RVOT in functional PR.

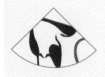

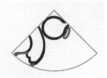

DTG RV 140°   ME RV in-out 60°   UE aortic arch SAX 90°

Leaflets
- Immobile or hypermobile cusps, dysplastic or hypoplastic cusps.
- Cusp flail is specific for severe PR.

Right heart
- RA and RV dilatation (Normal RV size excludes significant PR).
- Paradoxical septal motion from RV volume overload.

Colour Flow Doppler
- Retrograde diastolic jet towards to RVOT.
  - Duration of flow: may be a brief despite severe PR.
- Jet length poorly correlates with PR severity, Jet length > 10 mm sign of moderate PR.
- Jet width / RVOT ratio > 50 - 65% (sensitive sign, but low specificity for severe PR).
  - Diastolic flow reversal in main PA (100% sensitivity to detect severe PR, but also low specificity).
  - Vena contracta (VC) and EROA lacks validation trials.

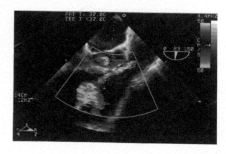

Severe PR in ME RV in-out view.

Spectral Doppler

- Good alignment UE Arch SAX and deep TG RV.
- Assessment of the flow velocity of PR.
  - Doppler trace shape and intensity indicates severity similar to AR.
  - PA ED pressure = $4 \times (PR_{ED})^2 + RAP$
  - mPAP = $4 \times (PR_{peak})^2 + RAP$
- Pressure half time (PHT): PHT < 100 ms = rapid deceleration (mid-diastolic termination of flow), which is consistent with severe PR.

12.4.2 Severity grading of PR

PARAMETERS	MILD	MODERATE	SEVERE
QUALITATIVE			
Valve morphology	Normal	Normal/abnormal	Abnormal
CF Doppler PR-jet	Small with narrow origin < 10mm	Intermediate	Large with wide origin May be brief in duration
PA flow reversal	Absent	Absent	Present
CW Doppler signal of PR-jet	Faint with slow deceleration	Variable/dense	Dense with early termination of diastolic flow
SEMI-QUANTITATIVE			
VC width	Not defined	Not defined	Not defined
PHT (ms)	Not defined	Not defined	< 100
Jet width ratio	Not defined	Not defined	> 50%
QUANTITATIVE			
EROA	Not defined	Not defined	Not defined
Regurg. Vol.	Not defined	Not defined	Not defined

12.5 Pulmonic stenosis

Pulmonic stenosis (PS) is a very rare disease.

Valvular	Congenital	Isolated	Dysplastic, unileaflet or bileaflet valve
		Associated with complex malformation	Tetralogy of Fallot, double outlet RV, univentricular heart
	Acquired	Infective endocarditis, carcinoid syndrome, rheumatic, tumor compression, prosthetic valve dysfunction	
Subvalvular	Congenital	RVOT obstruction in VSD	
	Acquired	Infiltrative disease, severe RV hypertrophy	
Supravalvular	Congenital	Rare	

12.6 Echocardiography

12.6.1 2D/3D TOE

- PV Morphology (numbers of leaflets, thickened leaflets, vegetations, calcification or systolic doming).
- RV Hypertrophy (RV WT > 5mm), and RV dilatation.
- Poststenotic PA dilatation (> 21 mm).
- Inspection of sub- and supravalvular area.
- Planimetry not feasible in 2D TOE.

- Antegrade turbulent flow at the level of obstruction and post-stenosis.
- Highest velocity must be used for severity assessment.
- Overestimation of gradients if concomitant PR.

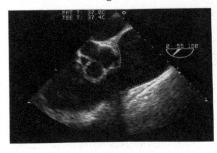

PS with severe poststenotic stenosis (dotted line).

Severity grading of PS

	TG PV	ME RV INFLOW-OUTFLOW	UE AORTIC ARCH SAX
2D imaging	Anterior cusp Annulus size	Left, anterior cusps Annulus size	Left, anterior cusps Annulus size
Colour flow Doppler (Nyquist 50-60cm/s)	PR (red) PS (turbulent)	PR (blue) PS (turbulent)	PR (blue) PS (turbulent)
Spectral Doppler	Good alignment	Poor alignment	Good alignment

PS	MILD	MODERATE	SEVERE
Peak velocity (m/s)	< 3	3 – 4	> 4
Peak gradient (mmHg)	< 36	36 – 64	> 64

12.7 References

1. Baumgartner H, et al.: Echocardiographic assessment of valve stenosis: EAE/ASE recommendations for clinical practice. J Am Soc Echocardiogr. (2009) 22:1-23; quiz 101-102.
2. Nicoara A, et al.: Guidelines for the Use of Transesophageal Echocardiography to Assist with Surgical Decision-Making in the Operating Room: A Surgery-Based Approach: From the American Society of Echocardiography in Collaboration with the Society of Cardiovascular Anesthesiologists and the Society of Thoracic Surgeons. J Am Soc Echocardiogr. (2020) 33:692-734.
3. Zoghbi WA, et al.: Recommendations for Noninvasive Evaluation of Native Valvular Regurgitation: A Report from the American Society of Echocardiography Developed in Collaboration with the Society for Cardiovascular Magnetic Resonance. J Am Soc Echocardiogr. (2017) 30:303-371.

13

Pericardial Pathology

JUSTIAAN SWANEVELDER
STEFAAN BOUCHEZ

13.1 Introduction

The pericardium is not essential and cardiac function can be normal in its absence. In about 1 on 35000 patients (0,003%) there is a partial or global absence of the pericardium. Usually pericardial fluid is not visible, with 15-50 ml ultrafiltrate fluid as normal.

The pericardium consists of
- An outer layer of parietal (and fibrous) pericardium.
- A serous, inner double-layer of visceral epicardium.

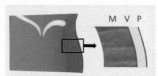

M, myocardium; V, visceral pericardium; P, parietal pericardium.

Function of the pericardium:
- Anatomic fixation of the heart preventing excessive motion.
- Provides mechanical protection to the heart.
- Barrier against infections.
- Reduces friction with the surrounding structures.

Pericardial sack attached to
- Great arteries: PA and aorta.
- Veins: superior vena cava (SVC), inferior vena cava (IVC) and 4 pulmonary veins.
- Two sinusses:
  - The transverse sinus: ME AV SAX and LAX.
  - The oblique sinus: ME AV LAX behind the left atrium.

ME AV LAX: green arrow indicates transverse sinus

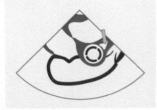

ME RV in-outflow: green arrow indicates transverse sinus

13.2 Pericardial effusions

13.2.1 Definition

An increase in the physiologic amount of pericardial fluid and associated
- With a minimal pericardial pressure increase.
- Without restriction of adequate filling of the heart.
- Without haemodynamic compromise.

13.2.2 Aetiology

- Idiopathic
- Infectious: viral, bacterial and parasitic
- Inflammation: post-AMI, uremia, post-surgical, systemic inflammatory disease (lupus, etc.).
- Traumatic: chest trauma, aortic dissection, postcatheter procedures, etc.
- Neoplasia: primary cardiac, metastatic, extension from lung or breast carcinoma.

13.2.3 Echocardiography

A pericardial effusion appears as an echo-free space between the two layers of the pericardium.
A pericardial effusion can be:
- Diffuse surrounding the heart.
- Loculated limited to one area of the pericardial space. Usually after surgical or percutaneous procedures.

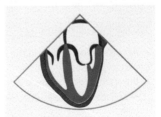

Effusion surrounding the heart (dark space)

PERICARDIAL EFFUSION	SEPARATION BY EFFUSION
Small	< 0,5 cm
Moderate	0,5 – 2 cm
Large	> 2 cm

Differential diagnosis with epicardial fat:
- Is also associated with other known factors, such as obesity, diabetes mellitus, age, hypertension and has been proposed as a marker of cardiovascular risk.
- Is identified as a hypoechoic and speckled space anteriorly to the RV, moving synchronously with the cardiac motions. The highest diameter is usually found on the RV free wall and the thickness should be measured in at least two locations.
- Echocardiographic measurements > 5 mm should define increased epicardial fat.

13.3 Cardiac tamponade

13.3.1 Definition

A cardiac tamponade is
- A clinical diagnosis in a haemodynamically unstable patient.
- A condition in which the pressure in the pericardial space is increased due to the accumulation of fluid or blood, resulting in haemodynamic abnormalities.
- A form of obstructive shock with clinical manifestations consistent with a low cardiac output and high RAP.

13.3.2 Pathophysiology

- Accumulation of fluid in the pericardial space → increased pericardial pressure.
- Intrapericardial pressure increase >> RV and LV filling pressures → collapse of cardiac chambers and haemodynamic deterioration.

2D TOE

- Pericardium: presence of a diffuse pericardial effusion and/or loculated collection of blood or fluid.
- RA systolic collapse.
  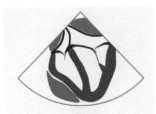
  Collapse of RA, RV and LA.
  - Because of the thin walled structure, brief RA collapse can occur even in the absence of tamponade.
  - The longer the duration of collapse relative to the cardiac cycle length, the greater the likelihood of tamponade.
  - Inversion greater than one third of the cardiac cycle has a sensitivity of 94% and a specificity of almost 100% for the diagnosis of tamponade.
- RV diastolic collapse.
  - occurs when pericardial pressure exceeds the RV diastolic pressure AND when RV wall is normal in thickness and compliance. Pre-existing PAH and RV hypertrophy will delay this finding. Occurs somewhat later than right atrial collapse in tamponade physiology.
  - This sign is higly specific (100%) for the diagnosis of tamponade.
- IVC dilatation and plethora.
  - a dilated IVC with < 50% inspiratory reduction in diameter is a sensitive (97%) but nonspecific (40%) indicator of tamponade. This finding reflects the elevated RAP.

Spectral Doppler

- Respiratory variation in diastolic filling.
    - Restrictive filling pattern.
    - Spontaneous inspiration: TV/PV peak velocities increase while MV E peak velocity and AV velocity increase.
    - IPPV: TV/PV velocities decrease, while MV/AV velocities increase. An excessive variation > 25% is observed.
- Tissue Doppler imaging.
    - Early diastolic mitral é is reduced in tamponade and returns to normal after pericardiocentesis.

13.4 Constrictive pericarditis

13.4.1 Definition

Fusion of the parietal and visceral pericardium leading to a scarred, thickened, often calcified pericardium, with resultant impairment of diastolic filling.

13.4.2 Aetiology

- Pericarditis.
- Cardiac surgery.
- Radiation therapy.
- Any other pericardial disease.

13.4.3 Pathophysiology

- Impaired diastolic filling due to rigid surrounding of the heart.
- Early diastolic filling is rapid with an abrupt cessation as diastolic pressure rises.
- The restricted filling leads to a fixed ED ventricular volume and fixed CO.
- Clinical signs: right-sided heart failure and low CO.

2D TOE
- Pericardium: increased echogenicity and thickening.
  - Normal pericardial thickness < 2mm.
  - Thickness > 3mm in 80% of patients with constrictive pericarditis.

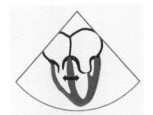

Thickened pericardium, dilated atria, paradoxical septal motion (arrow).

- Left ventricle:
  - Normal function.
  - Motion abnormalities.
    - IVS: respiratory variation.
    - Early diastole: abrupt posterior motion.
    - Mid diastole: flat motion.
    - Late diastole: anterior motion following atrial contraction.

  - Posterior wall
    - Flat pattern of diastolic posterior wall motion.
- Atria: "Mickey Mouse" appearance (both atria dilated) of the heart in ME 4C view is typical of chronic constrictive pericarditis.
- IVC dilatation.
  - This finding reflects the elevated RAP.

Spectral Doppler
- Respiratory variation in diastolic filling (PW Doppler).
  - Restrictive filling pattern.
  - Spontaneous inspiration: TV/PV peak velocities increase while MV E peak velocity and AV velocity increase.
  - IPPV: TV/PV velocities decrease, while MV/AV velocities increase. An excessive variation > 25% is observed.
- Hepatic vein Doppler using PW Doppler: reversal of diastolic flow during expiration.
- Tissue Doppler imaging.
  - S' > 8 cm/s.
  - Annulus reversus : mitral septal é (> 8 cm/s) > mitral lateral é (decreases with worsening constrictive pericarditis).
  - Annulus paradoxus: ratio E/é improves with worsening constrictive pericarditis.

13.5 Differentiation between restrictive pathologies

	NORMAL HEART	PERICARDIAL TAMPONADE	CONSTRICTIVE PERICARDITIS	RESTRICTIVE CARDIOMYOPATHY
ME 4C view				
Atria	Normal	Collapse (earliest RA)	Dilated	Dilated
Septal motion	Normal	Septal bounce	Septal bounce and septal cardiac shudder	No respiratory change
Transmitral flow	In / Ex	In / Ex	In / Ex	In / Ex
Spontaneous vent.	(E, A)	(E, A)	(E, A)	(E, A)
Mechanical vent.				
Hepatic vein Doppler	In / Ex	In / Ex	In / Ex	In / Ex
Spontaneous vent.	(S, D)	(S, D)	(S, Dr, A)	(S, D, A)
(Mechanical vent.: Vice versa)				

	NORMAL HEART	PERICARDIAL TAMPONADE	CONSTRICTIVE PERICARDITIS	RESTRICTIVE CARDIOMYOPATHY
TDI mitral S' cm/s	> 8	> 8	> 8	<< 8
TDI septal é cm/s	> 8 Lateral (<25%) > septal	< 8 Lateral > septal	> 8 Lateral ≤ septal	< 8 Lateral > septal
Ratio E/é	< 12	10 - 15 variable	< 15 Annulus paradoxus	> 15
GLS Strain pattern	Normal	Normal	'Hot' septum	Apical sparing

13.6 References

1. Little WC, et al. *Pericardial Disease*. Circulation (2006) 113:1622-1632
2. Chetrit M, et al. *Imaging-Guided Therapies for Pericardial Diseases, State-of-the-Art Review*. J Am Coll Cardiol Img. (2020) 13(6):1422–1437
3. Cosyns B, et al. *European Association of Cardiovascular Imaging (EACVI) position paper: multimodality imaging in pericardial disease*. Eur Heart J-Cardiovascular Imaging (2015) 16:12-31

14

Cardiac Masses

JOOST VAN DER MAATEN

14.1 Key points

- Cardiac pathologic masses are thrombus, vegetations or tumor.
- Signs and symptoms are nonspecific and highly variable related to the localization, size and composition of the cardiac mass.
- As echocardiography cannot give the histopathology, the rule of thumb for the differential diagnosis is:
  - Thrombus or vegetations are the most likely aetiology.
  - Primary cardiac tumors are mostly benign (most common are myxomas).
  - Metastatic tumors are the most common cardiac tumors.
  - Caveat: normal anatomic variants may mimic a cardiac mass.

14.2 Evaluation

The initial approach is to evaluate a mass in the clinical context. The next step is to consider whether this could be a:

a. Normal variant?
b. Thrombus or vegetation?
c. Metastasis?
d. Primary cardiac tumor?
e. Benign primary cardiac tumor?

14.3 Anatomical variants

Normal anatomic variants frequently mistaken for a pathologic mass:

Right atrium
- Eustachian valve: an embryologic remnant; originates at junction of IVC and RA; thin, filamentous and mobile structure.

- Chiari network: embryologic remnant; filamentous weblike structure in close relation to IVC and CS.
- Crista terminalis: muscle ridge that separates the smooth-walled RA from the trabeculated part, most prominent next to the SVC.
- Lipomatous hypertrophy of the interatrial septum: 'dumbell'-shaped fatty infiltration of the atrial septum, usually sparing the fossa ovalis.
- Interatrial septum aneurysm: prevalence 2-10%; mobile and redundant septum; associated with PFO.

Left atrial appendage (LAA)
- Pectinate muscles: muscular ridges in atria, most prominent in the LAA.
- Coumadin ridge: muscular ridge between the LAA and left upper pulmonary vein.

Right ventricle (RV)
- Trabeculations: muscle bands.
- Moderator band: echo-dense muscle band extending from the lower IVS across the RV cavity to the RV free wall.

Left ventricle (LV)
- Aberrant chordae tendinae: abnormal extra mitral valve chordae without structural function.
- False tendons: apically located thin strands running across the LV cavity.

Aortic valve
- Lambl's excrescences: thin, delicate filamentous strands that arise from the edge of the AV; normal degenerative process, seen increasingly with advancing age.

Tricuspid valve
- Annular fat: lipomatous thickening of the TV annulus.

Pericardium

- Cyst: small, rounded, echolucent mass, most often adjacent to the RA.

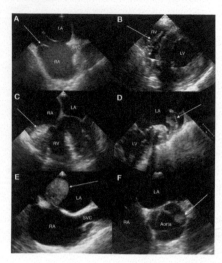

Examples of common cardiac masses. Eustachian valve (A), moderator band (B), TV annular fat (C), LAA thrombus (D), LA myxoma (E), AV papillary fibroelastoma (F).

14.4 Intracardiac thrombus or vegetation

14.4.1 Thrombus

- Irregular, homogenous mass of variable echogenicity.
- Thrombi move with underlying structure.
- Can be found in all cardiac chambers; LAA is most common location.
- Predisposing factors: atrial fibrillation, prosthetic valves, pacemaker wires and catheters, LV wall motion abnormalities (akinetic segments).

14.4.2 Vegetation

- See chapter on infective endocarditis.

14.5 Metastasis

- Metastatic tumors are the most common cardiac tumors.
- Typically involve the epicardium; pericardial effusion is common.
- Primary origin of metastasis is the lung (men) and breast (women).
- Melanoma has the highest rate of cardiac metastasis of all extra-cardiac tumors.

14.6 Primary cardiac tumors

14.6.1 Benign

- Primary cardiac tumors are mostly benign.
- Myxoma is the most common benign cardiac tumor in adults.
- Majority of myxoma (75–80%) is located in the LA.
- Characteristically originating from the mid-portion of the atrial septum by a narrow stalk attached to the fossa ovalis.
- Two basic appearances:
  - Polypoid myxomas: larger with a smooth surface and a rough core including lucencies and cystic areas; associated with atrioventricular valve obstruction and heart failure.
  - Papillary myxomas: smaller and irregular; associated with embolic phenomena.

14.6.2 Malignant

- Malignant primary cardiac tumors are rare, show a rapid grow invading cardiac structures (myocardium and pericardium).
- Most primary malignant cardiac tumors are sarcomas.
- When a cardiac tumor with features of malignancy on echocardiography is found, additional multimodality imaging is required.

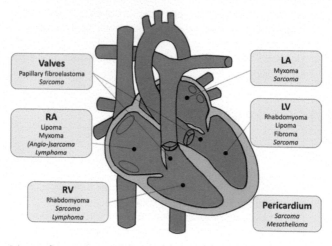

Valves
Papillary fibroelastoma
Sarcoma

LA
Myxoma
Sarcoma

RA
Lipoma
Myxoma
(Angio-)sarcoma
Lymphoma

LV
Rhabdomyoma
Lipoma
Fibroma
Sarcoma

RV
Rhabdomyoma
Sarcoma
Lymphoma

Pericardium
Sarcoma
Mesothelioma

Primary cardiac tumors by anatomic location.

14.7 References

1. Pepi M, et al. *European Association of Echocardiography. Recommendations for echocardiography use in the diagnosis and management of cardiac sources of embolism: European Association of Echocardiography (EAE) (a registered branch of the ESC)*. (2010) 11:461-476.
2. Galiuto L, et al. *The EAE Textbook of Echocardiography*. 1st edition. Oxford, Oxford University Press (2011)

15

Infective
Endocarditis

JOOST VAN DER MAATEN

15.1 Introduction

- Infective endocarditis (IE) is an uncommon but a potentially life-threatening infection of native and/or prosthetic valves associated with a high mortality.
- The modified Duke criteria are used as the primary diagnostic scheme.
- Complications occur in 50% of IE patients.
  - Valvular destruction causing heart failure.
  - Embolic events.
  - Perivalvular extension.

15.2 Echocardiography

15.2.1 Indications for echocardiography

- Echocardiography should be performed in all cases of suspected IE.
- TTE is recommended as the first-line imaging modality.
- TOE must be performed if high suspicion of IE because of:
  - Better image quality.
  - Better sensitivity.

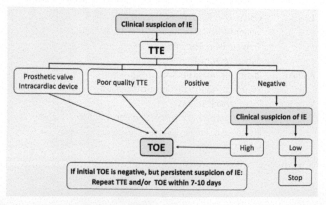

15.2.2 Limitations of echocardiography

- Sensitivity for IE, especially vegetations:

	NATIVE VALVES	PROSTHETIC VALVES
TTE	70	50
TOE	96	92

- Specificity for IE with TTE or TOE approximately 90%.
- Negative echo in 5-10% of cases of IE.
- Most difficult.
  - Small vegetations (<2mm).
  - Vegetations in the presence of pre-existent laesions (e.g. degenerative heart valves or prosthetic valves).
  - Intracardiac devices (e.g. pacemaker leads).

Vegetation	Oscillating or non-oscillating intracardiac mass or other endocardial structures or non-implanted intracardiac material
Abscess	Thickened non-homogeneous perivalvular area with echodense **or** echolucent appearance
Pseudoaneurysm	Pulsatile perivalvular echo-free space with CF Doppler detected
Perforation	Interruption of endocardial tissue continuity traversed by CF Doppler
Fistula	CF Doppler communication between 2 neighbouring cavities through a perforation
Valve aneurysm	Saccular bulging of valvular tissue
Dehiscence of a prosthetic valve	Paravalvular regurgitation identified by TTE/TOE with **or** without rocking motion of the prosthesis

Vegetation
- Definition:
  - A localized discrete mass.
    - Usually, irregular shape with sessile or peduncu- lated attachment.
    - At the upstream side of the valve or on prosthet- ic material.

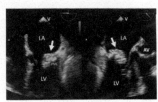

Vegetation

  - Moving back and forth during cardiac cycle.
  - The echodensity in early stages of IE is similar to soft tissue or thrombus.
- Predisposing conditions are BAV, valve degeneration, calcifica- tion and prosthetic valves.
- Progression of infection may result in leaflet perforation causing valvular regurgitation.
- Caveat
  - Aseptic vegetations may occur in non-bacterial thrombotic endocarditis (NBTE, also called marantic endocarditis, Lib- man-Sacks endocarditis).
  - Sterile vegetations on heart valves (mostly AV and MV).
  - Smaller and more prone to systemic embolization.
  - Located in the valvular coaptation lines .
  - Generally not accompanied by destruction of valvular tissue.
  - Associated with neoplasms or systemic autoimmune diseases (e.g. systemic lupus erythematosus).

- Risk of embolism
  - Risk of embolization increases with vegetation size and mobility.
  - MV vs AV involvement associated with increased risk of embolization.
  - In native or prosthetic AV and MV, vegetation size >10 mm is indication (class 1) for urgent surgery in symptomatic patients.
- Pitfalls
  - A variety of other findings may be mistaken for an infective vegetation:
    - Lambl's excrescences (delicate filamentous strands that arise from the edge of aortic valve leaflets).
    - Chordae tendineae.
    - Annular calcification (typically of MV annulus).
    - Myxomatous MV.
    - Eustachian valve or Chiari network.
    - Thrombus.
    - Sutures.
    - Other cardiac masses (e.g. fibroelastoma).
    - Beamwidth and side-lobe artefacts.

15.2.4 Perivalvular abscess

- Definition.
  - Thickened non-homogeneous perivalvular area with reduced echodensity *without* CF Doppler.
  - In early stage of tissue destruction only focal thickening of aortic wall may be seen.
  - More frequent in
    - Native AV IE.
    - Prosthetic valve IE.

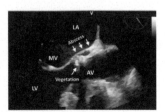

Peri-aortic valve abscess (white arrows) with echo-dense and echo-lucent appearance, and valvular regurgitation (MV, mitral valve; AV, aortic valve)

- Complications
  - Pseudoaneurysm
    - A pulsatile echo-free perivalvular space with CF Doppler.
  - Fistula
    - Tissue destruction resulting in perforation from aortic root abscess into the LV, RV, RA or LA.
    - Imaged with CF Doppler or CW Doppler (high-velocity flow).
  - Limitation of TOE.
    - TTE is more sensitive than TOE in detection of an anteriorly located abscess at the aortic septal junction.

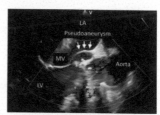

Pseudoaneurysm (white arrows) with colour flow in echo-lucent area.

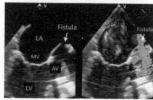

Fistula (white arrow) with colour flow between aortic root and left atrium.

15.2.5 New dehiscence of prosthetic valve

- Definition.
  - New perivalvular regurgitation.
  - Vegetation or abscess may be absent.

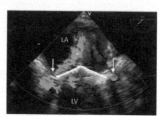

Perivalvular regurgitation (white arrows) of a mitral valve prosthesis (white lines represent prosthetic valve leaflets) with colour flow outside the prosthetic ring.

15.2.6 Right-sided and cardiac device related infective endocarditis (CDRIE)

- TV endocarditis commonly observed in IV drug users.
- Vegetations may be attached to atrial or ventricular side of the valve.
- PV is less frequently involved unless suspicion of congenital heart disease or intracardiac shunts.
- Permanent pacemaker leads are a risk factor.
- Most vegetations are attached to the leads; a smaller portion is attached to the TV.
- Artefacts of electrical wires may hamper identification of small vegetations.
- TOE is recommended in patients in suspected CDRIE with positive or negative blood cultures, independent of the results of TTE.

15.3 Echocardiographic indications for surgery

- Severe valvular regurgitation with signs of heart failure.
- Abscess.
- Large vegetation (>10mm).
- Prosthesis dehiscence.
- Increase in vegetation size despite appropriate antibiotic therapy.

15.4 References.

1. Habib G, et al. *Recommendations for the practice of echocardiography in infective endocarditis.* Eur J Echocardiogr. (2010) 11(2):202-219.
2. Habib G, et al. *ESC Guidelines for the management of infective endocarditis: The Task Force for the Management of Infective Endocarditis of the European Society of Cardiology (ESC). Endorsed by: European Association for Cardio-Thoracic Surgery (EACTS), the European Association of Nuclear Medicine (EANM).* Eur Heart J. (2015) 36(44): 3075-3128.

16

Artefacts and Pitfalls

JOACHIM ERB

16.1 Introduction

In general, imaging artefacts are the consequences of:
- Insufficient consideration of ultrasound physics.
- Inappropriate instrument setting.
- Inappropriate alignment of US-beam in regard to structure investigated.

Imaging artefacts cause the following results:
- Failure to visualize structures that are present.
- Make-believe structures that are not actually present, at least not in the imaged plane.
- Image of a structure differing in size and/or shape from the actual appearance.

Reasons for suboptimal image quality, needing exclusion first:
- Less than optimal imaging window to the heart.
- Air interface between transducer and structure visualized.
- Gastric contents in front of structure visualized.
- Angle between structure surface and ultrasound beam.

16.2 Echocardiography

16.2.1 2D - TOE imaging artefacts

Acoustic shadowing.
- Total reflection of the US beam occurs at tissue boundaries or structures with significant difference in acoustic impedance (density).
- US travel distal to this structure is blocked: calcification, air, prosthetic valve, cannula, tube.

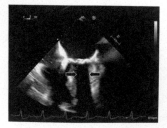

- Fan shaped shadow devoid of reflected signals along the direction of the scan line.
- Structures close to the transducer cast large shadows, peripheral structures, small shadows.

Reverberations – "Comet tail artefact" or "stepladder artefact"

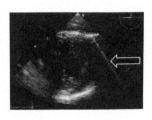

- Linear high amplitude echoes originating from two strong specular (= mirror) reflectors.
- US return to transducer is delayed by back-and-forth reflection between reflectors.
- Time delay mimics structures distal to the reflectors extending into the far field.
- Prominent reverberations can extinguish information from structures in the far field.

Side Lobe Artefacts

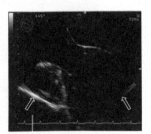

- Fractions of US energy are dispersed laterally from the main beam ($\sin \theta = n \lambda / D$).
- Strong specular (mirror) reflectors (i.e. calcifications, prosthetic material, catheters) produce echos if they are hit by the side lobes of neighboring US beams.
- The machine places the signal on the main beam → **double image**.
  - Arched lines extending laterally beyond the object in equidistance to the transducer.

Mirror Image Artefacts

- Conditions:
  - Good window, little interpositioned tissue.
    - Little attenuation of the ultrasound signal.
  - Strong, specular reflector in the near field.
    - Large amount of US energy is reflected, a part of which is reflected again at the transducer or a second specular reflector close to the transducer.
  - Depth setting ≥ 2 x distance between object and transducer.
    - US travels distance between object and transducer twice; equipment assumes reflection has originated from twice as far.
- Result: Mirror image at double distance from transducer.

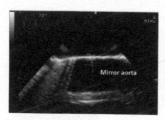
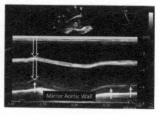

Air / gas interface artefact.

- Microbubbles of air / gas are very echogenic and cause multiple, bright dots on the image.
- Larger collections of air / gas appear as echogenic isles, but can also show as dark zones and cause a very characteristic mix of shadows and reverberation artefacts.
- Large air collections with a steady smooth blood / gas border cause total reflection of US, thereby acting as mirror reflectors causing double images.

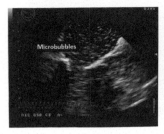
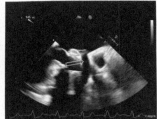

Low flow artefact.

- Slow moving blood increases its echogenicity and causes spontaneous echo contrast, which looks like whirling smoke.
- Very slowly moving or stagnating blood acts as ultrasound reflector and looks like a solid echogenic structure, similar to a thrombus.

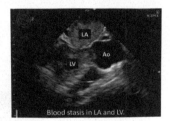

Blood stasis in LA and LV.

Electronic noise or interference.

- Erratic moving points or lines across the image in 2D, colour speckles with CF Doppler, for example with electrocautery (snowstorm).

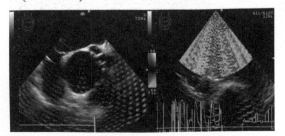

Aliasing.

- Limitation of maximal velocity correctly determined with PW and CF Doppler.
- Velocities above the threshold are depicted with the opposite sign.
- Inverse side of baseline (PW Doppler) or inverse colour (red vs blue) (CF Doppler).

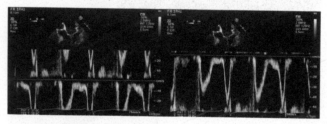

Nonparallel Beam Angle.

- Every degree in deviation from parallellism between blood flow and beam direction reduce the measured velocity by the factor cos α compared to the true velocity.

ANGLE α	20°	45°	60°	90°
Cosine α	0.94	0.71	0.5	0
Error in V	- 6 %	- 29 %	- 50 %	no results

Acoustic shadowing

- Beyond structures causing total ultrasound reflection, no signals can be collected.
  - No velocities and flow directions can be measured in the area of the US shadow.

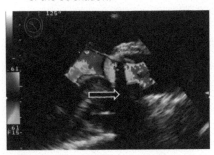

Mirror Image Artefacts

- Frequent with spectral Doppler if strong signals are recorded (low sample volume depth).
- Symmetric signal of lesser intensity in the opposite direction of the actual flow signal.
  - Upside down mirror image.
  - Can be reduced or eliminated by decreasing gain or power output at the instrument.

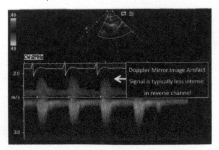

Range ambiguity – high PRF PW Doppler.
- High pulse repetition frequency Doppler allows multiplying the Nyquist limit by integer variables.
  - The number of measuring gates is multiplied by the same number.
  - Local discrimination difficult if additional gates contribute significant velocity readings.

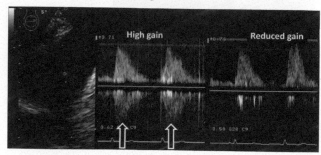

Ghosting artefact
- CF Doppler signals across the whole colour sector, even in areas with no flow due to moving strong reflectors in the image (mechanical valves).

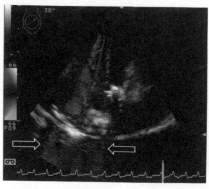

Air / gas interface artefact

- Microbubbles of air / gas are very echogenic and cause Doppler artefacts → colour speckles.
- Larger collections of air / gas can produce Doppler signals through resonance.
  - PW or CF Doppler signals.

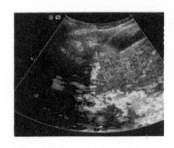

16.2.3 3D - TOE imaging artefacts

All artefacts known to regular 2D and Doppler imaging can appear in a 3D image.

In addition, there are the following artefacts genuine to 3D imaging.

Reconstruction (stitching) artefact

- With ECG-gated multiple beat image acquisition, movement (heart, patient, transducer by ventilation, arrhythmias) dislocates the structures slightly between heartbeats, to that the composed subvolumes show displacements at the interface due to incorrect juxtaposition.

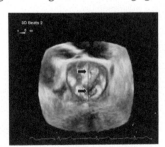

Dropout artefacts

- Weak or absent signals due to poor or little reflection lead to imaging dropout (lack of tissue often appearing as holes on valves or other thin structures, mainly IAS and AV).

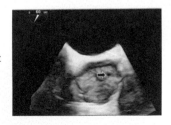

Blurring (Magnification) artefacts

- Thin, but echogenic structures appear thicker as they anatomically are because they act as strong reflectors in 3 dimensions with different resolutions. (e.g. MV chordae, sutures).

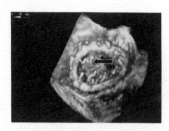

Blooming (star) artefact

- 3-dimensional side lobe artefacts caused by foreign bodies or highly echogenic structures producing fringes extending beyond the real structure like arrays – shining like a star.

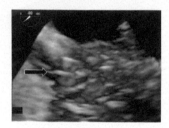

16.2.4 Pitfalls

Pitfalls are normal anatomical structures often mistaken or interpreted as pathology.

Structures commonly mistaken for thrombus, vegetation or tumor.

Crista Terminalis.

- Muscular ridge at the junction of RA and SVC separating the trabeculated RA appendage (RAA) from the smooth lined RA cavum.

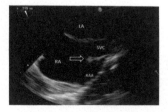

Eustachian Valve.

- Tissue rim at the transition of IVC into RA, as remnant of the embryologic valve directing IVC flow directly to the fossa ovalis.

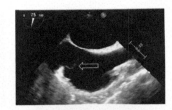

Chiari Network.

- Ribbon or net like fibers or fenestrated membranes which are embryonic remnants of sinus venosus valves, in close relation to IVC and CS.

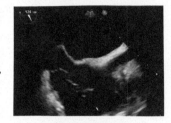

Thebesian Valve.

- Venous valve at the transition of the CS into the RA.

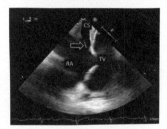

Moderator Band

(Trabecula septomarginalis).

- Tubular muscle running from the IVS to the free RV wall supporting it. It contains also conductive tissue.

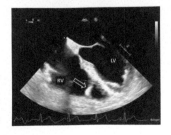

Lipomatous hypertrophy of the interatrial septum.
- Fatty infiltration usually sparing the fossa ovalis.

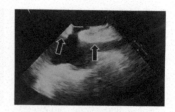

Coumadin Ridge.
- Also called warfarin ridge or left lateral ridge.
- Muscle ridge prone to lipomatous hypertrophy separating LAA and LUPV.

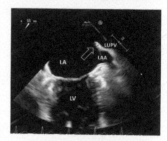

Noduli Arantii.
- Hyperplasia in the center of the free cusp margin of the AV, facilitating valve patency.

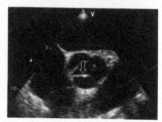

Lambl's excrescences.
- Benign filiforme irregularities at the free edges of the AV cusps close to the noduli Arantii.

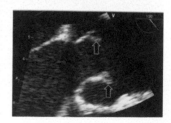

Apical mitral valve tendon.
- Accessory tendon inserting into the apical ventricular myocardium.

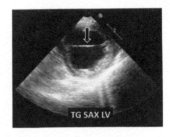

Structures commonly mistaken for cysts, passages or chambers.

Aneurysm of the interatrial septum.
- Floppy membrane, respective to actual PG between atria, bowing into one atrium or showing an oscillating motion between the atria.

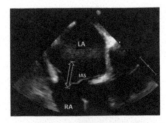

Pericardial sinuses.
- Pericardial folds, prone to misinterpretation when filled with pericardial fluid, blood or thrombus.
  - Transverse sinus: surrounding the origin of great vessels (Asc Ao, PA).
  - Oblique sinus: behind the left atrium and between the pulmonary vein entrance of both sides.

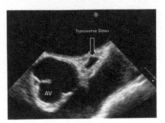

Other misinterpretations.

LPSVC (left persistent superior vena cava).
- Venous drainage from the left upper extremity connecting to the CS, running next to the LAA and left pulmonary veins (mistaken as cyst).

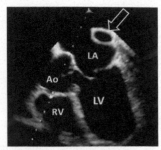

Hiatus hernia / Gastric fundus.
- Can be mistaken with the heart (LV) in the TG SAX view.

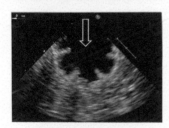

Pleural effusion.
- Mimicking aortic dissection on the left side.

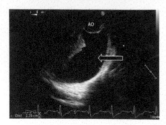

16.3 References.

1. Bertrand PB, et al. *Fact or Artefact in Two-Dimensional Echocardiography: Avoiding Misdiagnosis and Missed Diagnosis.* J Am Soc Echocardiogr. (2016) 29(5): 381-91.
2. Quien MM, et al. *Ultrasound imaging artefacts: How to recognize them and how to avoid them.* Echocardiography. (2018) 35(9): 1388-1401

17

Minimally Invasive Cardiac Surgery

STEFAAN BOUCHEZ

17.1 Introduction

17.1.1 Definition

Minimally invasive cardiac surgery (MICS) refers to the size of the incision, the avoidance of a sternotomy regardless the type of the surgical procedure. (In this chapter we mainly focus on cardio-pulmonary bypass (CPB)-related procedures although minimally invasive surgery also considers the avoidance of CPB).

17.1.2 Main indications

- Valve surgery: MV, TV, AV surgery.
- Tumor resection : myxoma, fibroelastoma etc.
- Correction of shunts: ASD, VSD etc.

17.1.3 Contraindications

- Contraindication for TOE.
- Severe aortic disease: aortic dissection, > grade 3 atherosclerosis, ascending aorta dilatation > 40 mm.
- Absence of the SVC or IVC.
- Congenital RA /RV outflow tract obstruction: thrombus.

17.2 Echocardiography

17.2.1 Pre-CPB

First phase
- A complete TOE exam with specific attention for
  - PFO:
    - Need for bicaval cannulation.
    - Risk for air embolism.
    - Risk for perioperative flooding of the operating field.

- Left pleural effusion.
  ◦ Impact on left single lung ventilation.
- Detailed description of the surgical pathology.

Second phase
- Positioning of guidewires and cannulas.
  - Complications: perforation and bleeding.
- Central venous line insertion.
  - ME bicaval view: position of guidewire and catheter.
- Coronary sinus catheter.
  - Installed for the admin- istration of cardioplegia if antegrade cardioplegia administration is not feasible.
  - ME bicaval view: introduc- tion of catheter.
  - Correct positioning: TG Basal SAX with the CS above the basal MV.

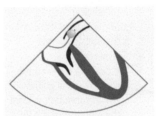

- Cannulation of the SVC by the anaesthesiologist.
  - Depending on the needs of the surgeon, one or two venous cannulas may be placed. Most commonly one venous cannula is placed into SVC and an- other into the IVC. When access to the RA is necessary, two cannulas are always used.

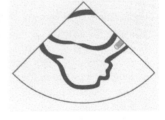

  - First a guidewire is inserted into the jugular vein and advanced until echocardiographic confirmation of its proper position in the SVC in the ME bicaval view.

- The cannula is then advanced over the guidewire into the SVC and its position should not exceed the junction of the RA and the SVC.
- Cannulation of the IVC by the surgeon.
  - A guidewire is introduced into the femoral vein under direct vision by the surgeon and advanced until echocardiographic confirmation of its position in the SVC in the ME bicaval view.

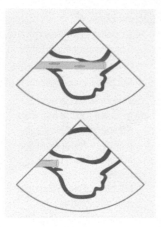

  - The cannula is than advanced over the guidewire.
    ○ Single cannulation: until the junction of the RA and the SVC.
    ○ Bicaval cannulation: until the junction of the RA and the IVC.
- Cannulation of the femoral artery by the surgeon.
  - A guidewire is introduced into the femoral artery under direct vision by the surgeon and its position in the descending aorta is confirmed in the ME desc Ao SAX. Once confirmed, the surgeon will introduce the cannula over the guidewire.

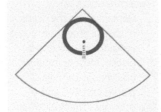

- Introduction of the endo-aortic balloon (EAB).
  - Another guidewire is advanced through the hemostatic valve of the lateral port of the femoral cannula. Again, the guidewire must be visualized in the descending aorta and followed into the arch and the aortic root.
  - In the ME AV LAX view, the EAB is slowly advanced until the STJ is reached. The final positioning and insufflation of the EAB will be performed after the start of CPB.

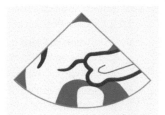

17.2.2 During CPB

Monitoring adequate position of cannulas.
- Check for dissection at start of CPB (peripheral arterial femoral access).
  - Pseudodissection versus true dissection.
    - Upon initiation of CPB of peripheral CPB, the separation of flows (blood versus priming fluids) gives a pseudodissection appearance to the aorta.

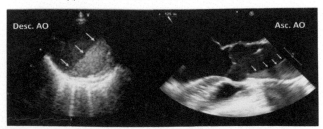

Desc. AO   Asc. AO

Pseudodissection (yellow arrows)

- EAB catheter insufflation and positioning.
  - ME LAX view: Position of the EAB at the STJ.
    - No inflation of EAB if not (properly) visible.
    - Adenosine administration before insufflation of EAB to obtain a cardiac standstill.
  - Continuous monitoring of the position before, during and immediately after the administration of cardioplegia is obligatory as pressure changes in the aortic root may cause displacement of the EAB. Displacement of the EAB:
    - Too proximal:
      › Cardioplegia ineffective as the EAB obstructs the coronary arteries.
      › May cause AR.
    - Too distal:
      › Right radial artery damping.
      › May impair cerebral perfusion.

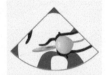
EAB too proximal.

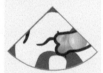
EAB in correct position

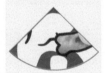
EAB too distal.

– The flow of the cardioplegia can be visualized by CF Doppler. With adequate cardioplegia delivery, also the low flow ('smoke') pattern present in the aortic root will rapidly disappear.

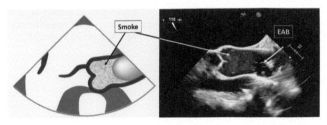

– Once the LA is opened, the echocardiographic window will usually disappear, and the visualization of the ascending aorta will become very difficult. Therefore, ensure a proper position of the EAB before the surgeon opens the LA.

17.2.3 Post CPB

- After unclamping the presence of air in the LA and LV must be evaluated. Always check for RWMA of the LV during and after CPB, especially in MV surgery (Cx art.). Adequate deairing is more difficult in MICS, but carbon dioxide insufflation promotes rapid resorption. Sometimes air/carbon dioxide can be visualized in the ascending aorta when the heart is not yet fully ejecting while on peripheral CPB.
- Confirmation of adequacy of surgical result.
- Haemodynamic assessment before coming of CPB.

17.3 References

1. Coddens J, et al. *Transesophageal echocardiography for port-access surgery*. J Cardiothorac Vasc Anesth 1999; 13: 614 – 622

2. Lebon JS, et al. *Transesophageal echocardiography for minimally invasive cardiac surgery*. Transesophageal Echocardiography – Multimedia Manual. (2nd ed.) editors Denault A., Couture P., Vegas A., Buithieu J., Tardif JC. Informa Healthcare UK. 2011; 511 - 527

18

Fluid Status
Evaluation

R. F. TRAUZEDDEL
C. BERGER
S. TRESKATSCH

18.1 Introduction

- Fluid status can be evaluated using static and dynamic parameter.
  - Static parameters:
    - LV EDA.
    - Ratio of RV and LV dimensions (RV/LV index).
    - Kissing papillary muscle sign (KPMS).
    - Position of the interatrial septum.
  - Dynamic parameters:
    - SVC collapsibility index (SVC-CI).
    - IVC distensibility index (SVC-DI) (more applicable in TTE).
    - Passive leg raising test.
    - SV variation (SVV).
- Always take possible previous echocardiographic as well as clinical findings into account and compare them with the current examination.
- Fluid status evaluation with static parameters is only feasible in absence of reduction in pulmonary blood flow (e.g. hypoxic pulmonary vasoconstriction, pulmonary embolism).
- LV SVV cannot be used in severe heart rhythm disturbances (e.g. atrial fibrillation), RV dysfunction and low tidal volume.

18.2 Echocardiography

18.2.1 Static parameters

LV end-diastolic area
- Measured in TG Mid SAX at ED.
- Indication of hypovolemia if LV EDA < 5.5 cm²/m² BSA.
  - Exclusion: LV Hypertrophy ++ (LV septal WT > 14 mm).
- Cave: Preoperative dilated LV with reduced EF + normal LV EDA = hypovolemia.

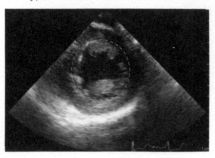

RV/LV index
- Measured in ME4C at ED (basal to midventricular region)
- LV filling depends on the preload provided by RV.
  - RV failure will cause LV hypovolemia.

- Achieved visually with the help of the volume/diameter relation between RV and LV.
- RV/LV-Index:
  - normal ratio is ~ 0.6
  - RV/LV-Index $\geq$ 1.0 indicates severe RV dilatation.

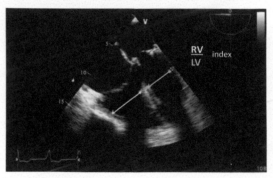

Kissing papillary muscle sign
- Sign best witnessed during systole in TG Mid SAX at the level of the PM reflecting a very low LV ES area (LV ESA).
- Opposite myocardial walls of associated ventricle come into contact with one another.
- Important to measure LV EDA (see section under LV EDA to differentiate low SVR states from hypovolemia.
  - Normal LV EDA + KPMS suggestive of low SVR.

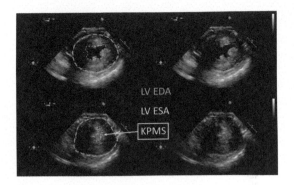

Position of the interatrial septum (IAS)

- With regard to atrial volume status, a visual assessment of IAS in the ME 4C or bicaval view can be used for qualitative estimation of atrial filling pressures.
- Hypermobile IAS during states of low bi-atrial filling such as during global hypovolemia (Cave: IAS aneurysm has to be excluded).
- IAS permanently convex to RA indicates increased LAP.
  IAS permanently convex to LA in combination with LV hypo-volemia indicates increased RAP.
  IAS fixed in the middle in context of global hypervolemia with all heart chambers appearing "overfilled" or "stretched".

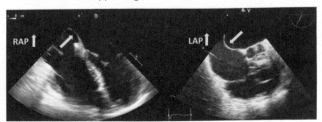

18.2.2 Dynamic parameters

Superior vena cava collapse index (SVC-CI)
- Measured in the ME bicaval view in supine position.
- Due to intrathoracic position SVC will be compressed during mechanical inspiration (collapse).
- The more pronounced the intravascular hypovolemia, the greater the SVC collapsibility, thus the greater the volume responsiveness.
- SVC-CI = $100 \times (SVC_{exsp} - SVC_{insp})/SVC_{exsp}$
- SVC-CI > 36% indicates positive volume responsiveness in mechanically ventilated, septic patients.

Qualitative echocardiographic evaluation of volume status / fluid responsiveness.

STATUS	RESPIRATORY MODULATION	INTERPRETATION	FLUID RESPONSIVENESS
SVC dilated (*i.e. round in shape, stretched, visual aspect of overfilling*)	No variation	Filling pressure ↑	Negative (*"Stop signal" for further fluid administration*) *
SVC small/collapsed	Pronounced variation	Filling pressure ↓	Positive
SVC intermediate	Passive Leg Raising (PLR) and/or Fluid challenge (FC) If SV increases with unchanged SVR, fluid substitution is clinically indicated.		

* In the context of chronic cardiovascular disease, a positive volume responsiveness may occasionally be given despite a dilated SVC without respiratory oscillation. Further evaluation may be done by means of PLR/FC.

Stroke volume (SV) in the LV outflow tract (LVOT)

- SV assessesment by VTI_{LVOT} and CSA_{LVOT} : see chapter on haemo-dynamic monitoring.
- Mechanical ventilation induced changes induce SV variation (SVV).
  - SV correlates with VTI_{LVOT} and LVOT velocity (V_{LVOT}) as the LVOT diameter remains the same in each patient.
    - End of inspiration: decrease of SV, VTI_{LVOT} and V_{LVOT} (depressed RV preload & ejection)
    - End of expiration : increase of SV, VTI_{LVOT} and V_{LVOT}.
  - The minimum and maximum V_{LVOT} can easily be recorded by PW Doppler in the ME LAX or TG LAX view. ΔV_{LVOT} is calculated as the percentage change in peak V_{LVOT} in one respiratory cycle.
    - $$\Delta V_{LVOT} = \frac{V_{LVOTmax} - V_{LVOTmin}}{(V_{LVOTmax} + V_{LVOTmin})/2} \times 100$$
  - An increased SVV (> 11 %) is a predictor of fluid responsiveness under mechanical ventilation in the absence of RV failure or rhythm disturbances.

18.3 References

1. Trauzeddel R.F., *et al. Perioperative echocardiography-guided hemodynamic therapy in high-risk patients: a practical expert approach of hemodynamically focused echocardiography.* J Clin Monit Comput. (2021) 35(2):229-243.
2. Miller A, et al. *Predicting and measuring fluid responsiveness with echocardiography.* Echo Res Pract. (2016) 3(2):G1-G12.

19

Haemodynamic Monitoring

NICK FLETCHER

19.1 Introduction

Echocardiography can be used to assess many aspects of circulatory function in the cardiac theatre and critical care unit. A good clinician should integrate examination and information from other monitors.

19.2 Echocardiography

19.2.1 Right atrial pressure (RAP)

- Estimation of RAP by evaluating the size and degree of collapse of the IVC.
- Measured 1 cm from the diaphragm in the IVC view.
- These values are validated in spontaneously breathing patients.

RAP mmHg	IVC SIZE IN CM	DEGREE OF IVC COLLAPSE
5	<2	>50 %
10	2	<50 %
15	>2	<50 %

- Note that this is a static measurement. Dynamic assessment of fluid responsiveness may also be assessed from the IVC reactivity in spontaneous and controlled breathing.

19.2.2 Right ventricular systolic pressure (RVSP) / Systolic pulmonary artery pressure (sPAP)

- CF Doppler to visualize TR in the modified ME bicaval view or other RA views.
- Use CW Doppler to measure the regurgitant velocity.

- Peak regurgitant velocity can be used to estimate the gradient between the RV and the RA with the use of the simplified Bernouilli equation:
  - RV Gradient (mmHg) = 4 x (peak velocity TR)^2
  - RVSP = RV Gradient + RAP mmHg
  - Normal assumption is no gradient over the PV, so the RVSP equals sPAP.
  - RVSP = sPAP

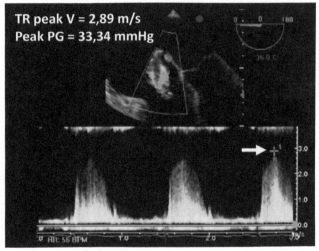

RV Gradient in this example = 33 mmHg
RAP via invasive pressure measurement = 13 mmHg
sPAP is 33 + 13 = 46 mmHg

19.2.3 Mean pulmonary artery pressure (mPAP)

4 methods to estimate mPAP:

1. From sPAP:
   mPAP mmHg = 0,61 x sPAP + 2
2. From VTI of TR: by tracing the CW Doppler contour of TR.
   mPAP mmHg = VTI_{TR} + RAP
3. From PR: measuring peak velocity of PR.
   mPAP = peak PR velocity + RAP
4. From the pulmonary acceleration time (pACT)
   Measure pACT using PW Doppler.
   – Normal pACT (normal PA-pressures): > 120 msec
   – mPAP = 79 – (0,45 x pACT)

2 methods to estimate LAP:

1/ From MR in the ME 4C view.
- Peak MR velocity can be used to estimate the gradient between the LV and the LA with the use of the simplified Bernouilli equation: LV Gradient (mmHg) = 4 x (peak velocity MR)^2
- In the absence of AS, LV systolic pressure equals systolic blood pressure (BP$_{sys}$): LAP = LV Gradient – BP$_{sys}$

2/ From TDI and transmitral spectral Doppler in the ME 4C view.
- Measure transmitral E velocity using PW Doppler.
- Measure lateral é using TDI.
- The ratio of E/é gives a good estimate of LAP:
  - Formula by Nagueh: 1,24 x (E/é + 1,9)
  - Simplified formula: LAP = E/é + 4

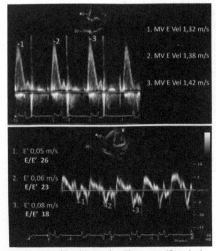

Measurements of E and E'. Note how E' can vary with respiration due to physiological changes and variation of Doppler placement

19.2.5 Stroke volume and cardiac output measurement

Stroke volume (SV) can be calculated on the LV (using LVOT) or on the RV (using RVOT).

- First measure LVOT diameter (D_{LVOT}) in the ME LAX or ME AV LAX view.
  - The cross-sectional area (CSA) of the LVOT is calculated with the formula $\pi \times r^2$.
  - Since the radius r = Diameter/2 this formula can be rephrased:
    - CSA = $\pi \times r^2$
    - CSA = $\pi / 4 \times D_{LVOT}^2$
    - **CSA = 0,785 x D_{LVOT}^2**
- Next measure LVOT flow in the Deep TG or TG LAX view.
  - Measure VTI_{LVOT} by tracing the LVOT Doppler contour.
  - The VTI or stroke distance is measured in cm. The CSA multiplied by the stroke distance provides a SV.

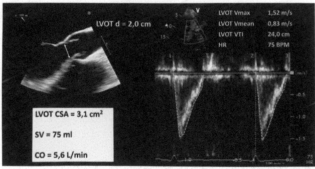

$SV = SV = VTI_{LVOT} \; x \; CSA_{LVOT}$
$CO = Heart \; rate \; (HR) \; x \; SV$

19.3 Case

A 77 year old man having CABG. His BSA is 2 m^2.

VITALS & TOE:			CALCULATE:
Heart rate	75 bpm	1/	Stroke volume (SV)
Arterial BP	105/65 mmHg	2/	Cardiac output (CO)
RAP	10 mmHg	3/	Cardiac index (CI)
Diameter LVOT	2,2 cm	4/	Systolic pulmonary artery pressure (sPAP)
TVI LVOT	18 cm	5/	Mean pulmonary artery pressure (mPAP)
Peak velocity LVOT	1 m/s	6/	Left atrial pressure (LAP)
Peak velocity TR	2,8 m/s		
Pulmonary ACT	128 msec		
Mitral valve E velocity	0,94 m/s		
TDI lateral é	0,12 m/s		

Answers:

1/ SV = VTI_{LVOT} x CSA_{LVOT} = 18 x 3,8 = 68 ml

2/ CO = SV x HR = 68 x 75 = 5,1 L/min

3/ CI = CO/BSA = 5,1/2 = 2,6 L/min/m^2

4/ sPAP:

RVSP = 4 x TR^2 = 31 mmHg

sPAP = RVSP + RAP = 31 + 10 = 41 mmHg

5/ mPAP:
 - Using sPAP = 0,61 x sPAP +2 = 21 mmHg
 - Using pACT = 79 – (0,45 x pACT) = 21 mmHg

6/ LAP:
 - Nagueh: 1,24 x (0,45 x E/é) = 12 mmHg
 - Simplified formula: E/é + 4 = 12 mmHg

19.4 References

1   Nicoara A, et al. *Guidelines for the Use of Transesophageal Echocardiography to Assist with Surgical Decision-Making in the Operating Room: A Surgery-Based Approach: From the American Society of Echocardiography in Collaboration with the Society of Cardiovascular Anesthesiologists and the Society of Thoracic Surgeons.* J Am Soc Echocardiogr (2020) 33(6): 692-734.

2. Geisen M, et al. *Echocardiography-based hemodynamic management in the cardiac surgical intensive care unit.* J Cardiothorac Vasc Anesth (2014) 28(3): 733-44.

3. Vieillard-Baron A, et al. *Diagnostic workup, etiologies and management of acute right ventricle failure: A state-of-the-art paper.* Intensive Care Med (2018) 44(6): 774-90.

20

Congenital Heart Disease

DOMINIQUE BETTEX
PIERRE-GUY CHASSOT

20.1 Introduction

Congenital heart diseases (CHD) occur in 0.5-1% of living births. Complex heart malformations represent only 0.15% of living births. Nowadays, the majority of children with congenital disease are reaching adulthood, so that the population of adults with CHD or GUCH grown-up congenital disease (GUCH) is slowly becoming larger than the pediatric one.

CONGENITAL HEART DEFECT	PREVALENCE IN LIVE BIRTHS %	PROPORTION OF CHD %
Ventricular septal defect	0,25	30,0
Atrial septal defect	0,15	20,0
Patent ductus arteriosus	0,09	10,0
Pulmonic stenosis	0,05	5,0
Persistent left vena cava	0,05	5,0
Tetralogy of Fallot	0,04	3,5
Coarctation aortae	0,04	3,5
Transposition of great arteries	0,03	3,0

20.2 Echocardiography

20.2.1 Persistent Left Superior Vena Cava (PLSVC)

Pathophysiology

The LSVC drains into CS. Attention is required with left-sided catheterization and during cardiac surgery (cannulation and surgical repair). The dilated CS may compress conduction tissues, leading to arrhythmias.

Echocardiography

- Dilated CS in ME 4-chamber (0°), 2-chamber (90°), TG Basal SAX or at the transition between TG Basal SAX and the ME 4C view.
- Intravenous injection of agitated saline into the left sided vein opacifies the CS.

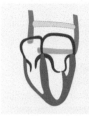

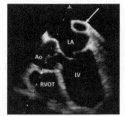

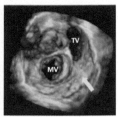

Anatomy (one variant)   *ME 4C: dilated CS (arrow)*   *surgical view of MV and severely dilated CS (arrow)*

20.2.2 Atrial septum defect (ASD)

Pathophysiology

Left to right shunt leading to RV volume overload with RA and RV dilatation. This predisposes to arrhythmias and a progressive increase in PVR in some patients. Risk of paradoxical emboli.

Four types:

1. Ostium secundum: most common type in 75% of ASD.
2. Ostium primum: within the spectrum of AVSD (atrio-ventricular septum defect) in 15% of ASD.
3. Sinus venosus: two types, superior > inferior. In 9% of ASD. The superior type is frequently associated with partial anomalous pulmonary venous return (PAPVR).
4. CS unroofing: almost always associated with a LSVC.

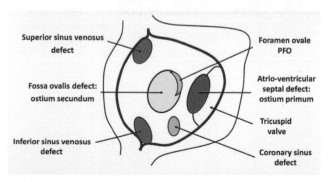

Echocardiography

PATHOLOGY	PFO	ASD I	ASD II	SINUS VENOSUS ASD
TOE scanplanes	ME 4C ME AV SAX ME Bicaval	ME 4C TG Basal SAX	ME 4C ME AV SAX ME Bicaval	ME Bicaval (SVC/IVC)
Defect	No tissue defect, but tissue flap in IAS	Tissue defect in lower portion of IAS, immediately adjacent to the AV valves	Tissue defect within the fossa ovalis (center IAS)	Tissue defect in upper (SVC) or lower (IVC) part of IAS.
Associations	Interatrial septum aneurysm	Cleft MV, inlet VSD	MV proplapse, Ebstein's anomaly	PAPVD usually of right PV
2D	Localisation of ASD including number, size and form of the orifices. Use of a bubble test in case of PFO. Measurements of length of rims. Associated RA and RV dilatation, PA proportional to the dimension and duration of defect(s)			
CF Flow	Direction of shunt flow, laminar if large or mildly turbulent if small. Check pulmonary venous return and associated valvular regurgitation			
Spectral Doppler	Direction of flow: usually L-R shunt with short period of R-L shunt during early systole and mid-diastole. PW Doppler over ASD shows low velocity (max < 1,5 m/s) predominantly during diastole. Quantification of shunt.			
3D	Confirm findings using 3D and 3D CF Doppler			

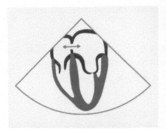

ASD II defect in fossa ovalis.

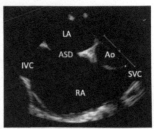

ASD II in modified 2D ME bicaval view (arrow)

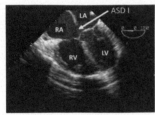

ASD I with septum primum defect (arrow)

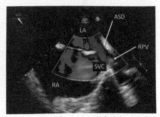

Sinus venosus defect with RPV draining into SVC

ASD shunt quantification

- $Qp/Qs = \dfrac{(CSA_p \times V_p max)}{(CSA_{ao} \times V_{ao} max)} \geq 1.5$ requires correction

  (p pulmonary artery, ao Aorta)

TOE sequence for the evaluation of ASD

1. Localization of ASD including number, size and form of the orifices.
2. Length of the rims.
3. Pulmonary venous return.
4. Direction of the shunt.
5. Quantification of the shunt: Qp/Qs.
6. After closure, exclude residual shunt, pulmonary venous stenosis (sinus venosus type).
7. Exclude device impingement on surrounding anatomic structures.
8. Exclude pericardial effusion, thrombus, device embolization.

20.2.3 Patent foramen ovale (PFO)

Pathophysiology

Paradoxical emboli due to shunting. A PFO of > 4 mm on TOE has been associated with a greater risk for stroke. The incidence (based on autopsy) is estimated at > 30 % of population.

Echocardiography

- 2D: ME 4C, ME AV SAX or ME bicaval view.
- CF Doppler: set scale at 30 cm/s to optimize the visualization of flow in PFO.
- Bubble test under Valsalva-release:
  - Efficacy of Valsalva = defined by a 20 cm/s decrease in trans-mitral E velocity.
  - Use of agitated saline: a mixture of 8 ml saline with 1 ml air and 1 ml of blood may be better than saline and air alone.
  - > 5 bubbles from R → L during the next 3 cardiac cycles after right opacification.
  - Intrapulmonary shunts when bubbles appear on the left side after > 5 cardiac cycles.
- PFO closure device: assess size, localization, correct closure, absence of device impingement on surrounding structures and look for the presence of pericardial fluid in case of interventional closure.

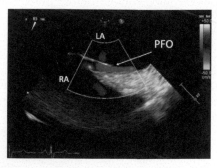

ME AV SAX: CF Doppler through PFO

20.2.4 Ventricular Septum Defect (VSD)

Pathophysiology.
Paradoxical emboli due to shunting, RV and LV overload, PA
overflow.

Four types
- Membranous or perimembranous VSD (70%).
- Muscular or trabecular VSD (20%).
- Inlet VSD or AV-canal type: associated with AVSD (5%).
- Supracristal, infundibular, subarterial or outlet VSD (5%).

Echocardiography

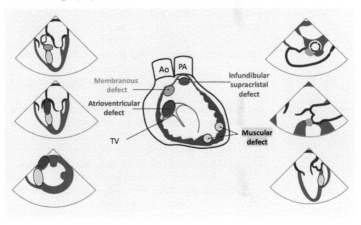

VENTRICLE SEPTUM DEFECT (VSD)	PERIMEMBRA-NOUS	MUSCULAR	INLET	OUTLET
TOE scan planes	ME 4C ME AV SAX ME (AV) LAX ME RV In - Out	Deep TG TG Mid SAX ME 4C	TG Mid SAX ME 4C	ME RV In - Out
Location	Membranous septum, inferomedial to AV and lateral to TV septal leaflet	Muscular septum central or apical Mostly antero-apical	Inferior to AV and close to both TV and MV	RV outflow tract below AV and near the PV
Associations	AV (RCC) herniation and AR, subaortic stenosis	Acquired after AMI	Straddling chordae from septal TV to LV	AV (RCC) herniation
2D	Location, type and size of VSD. RV, LV, LA, PA dimensions related to size of defect. RV and LV function (volume overload). Valvular pathology TV, AV, MV.			
CF Doppler	Direction of shunt flow (L → R, bidirectional). Laminar flow is large VSD, mostly turbulent. Turbulences within the RV. Flow convergence (PISA) on LV. Asses valvular dysfunction: AR, MR and TR.			
Spectral Doppler	Direction of flow: usually L-R or bidirectional (=Eisenmenger). Restrictive versus non-restrictive VSD. Calculation of RVSP: SBP – VSD-gradient where VSD-gradient= $4 \times V_{VSD}^2$ Quantification of shunt Qp/Qs			
3D	Confirm findings using 3D and 3D CF Doppler			

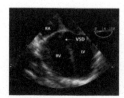

Perimembranous VSD

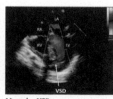

Muscular VSD

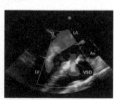

Supracristal VSD

VSD shunt quantification

- $Qp/Qs = Qp/Qs = \dfrac{(CSA_p \times V_p max)}{(CSA_{ao} \times V_{ao} max)}$

  (*p pulmonary artery, ao Aorta*)

TOE sequence for the evaluation of VSD

1. Localization (perimembranous, supracristal, inlet, muscular).
2. Size, number and form of the defect.
3. Direction of the shunt.
4. Assessment of adjacent structures.
5. Quantification of the shunt: Qp/Qs.
6. 3D guidance for interventional closure of VSD.
7. After closure, assess residual shunts, PA pressures, RV and LV function, AR, TR, LVOTO, RVOTO.
   - Residual VSD: residual VSD < 2mm will generally close spontaneously; ≤ 3 mm generally haemodynamically not significant. If large residual defect (≥ 4 mm or Qp/Qs > 1.5/1) with flow convergence on the LV side, discuss re-intervention.
   - TR in case of tethering or partial disinsertion.
   - AR after supracristal VSD closure.
   - Look for RVOTO unmasked after closure of the VSD.
   - In case of multiple VSD, look for new apparition of preexistant muscular VSD after closure of the largest ones.

20.2.5 Fontan circulation

Pathophysiology
Circulatory flow depends on adequate transpulmonary flow. The goals are to keep pulmonary pressures low and systemic ventricular function adequate.

Rerouting of the systemic venous return directly into the PA thereby bypassing the right heart, was first described by Fontan in 1971: atrio-pulmonary anastomosis. Nowadays, a bidirectional Glenn anastomosis (end-to-side anastomosis of the SVC to the right PA) acts as a staging procedure followed by the complete rerouting of the venous return through an internal tunnel from IVC to PA, or through a conduit (FC) between IVC and PA.

Fontan haemodynamics:

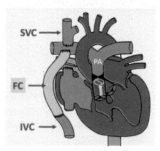

- Elimination of the mixing of the systemic and pulmonary venous blood and relief of the cyanosis while suppressing the volume load on the single ventricle by restoring a circulation in series.
- Preload of the ventricle is an important determinant for the circulatory output and is determined mainly by the transpulmonary flow. The transpulmonary flow drive relies on the PG between RAP and LAP (gradient of 6-10 mmHg considered necessary) and the PVR.
- Haemodynamic goal: promote forward flow over the lungs by avoiding increases in PA-pressures and atrial pressure.

Echocardiography
2D TOE
- Systemic ventricle: (standard references are not available).
  - Dimensions.
  - Systolic function.
  - Diastolic function: impaired diastolic function is common in single ventricles despite preserved systolic function.
- Atrioventricular valve.
  - Morphology including structural abnormalities.
- Fontan and anastomoses.
  - Modified ME Bicaval, ME Asc Ao LAX and UE Ao Arch SAX views for the assessement of the SVC and IVC anastomoses.
- Aortic outflow tract obstruction or AS: the relation between the systemic ventricle and the aortic tract is variable. Often the flow crosses a VSD or bulboventricular foramen which may cause flow restriction and functions as a subaortic stenosis. Assess also for the presence of LVOTO and AS.

Colour Flow Doppler
- Atrioventricular valve: regurgitation is a common long-term complication in single ventricle physiology. There are no specific guidelines for the assessment of systemic valve regurgitation, the principles outlined in the guidelines may be applied.
- Flow through fenestration at the level of the atrium: shunting is always right to left reflecting the systemic venous hypertension.
- Fontan flow and flow at anastomoses: Flow should be laminar.

Spectral Doppler

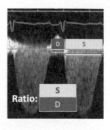

- Ventricular function: the determination of the systolic to diastolic duration ratio can be used to assess the RV function (Hypoplastic Left Heart Syndrome) using atrioventricular regurgitation duration from Doppler flow. Ventricular dysfunction was considered in patients with a S/D duration ratio > 2.

- Flow profile (Doppler) through the veno-pulmonary anastomosis:
  - Normal: biphasic forward flow with peak velocities during systole and diastole of 0.2 to 0.5 m/sec or forward flow with flow reversals.
  - Obstruction: A high flow velocity (> 1.5 m/s), without cyclic variations, and not reaching baseline during cardiac and/or respiratory cycle, is suggestive of a significant obstruction.
  - Ventilatory-induced changes in flow: flow attenuation or even reversal during the positive-pressure phase of IPPV. Maximal flow during spontaneous inspiration.

- Fontan fenestration: PW Doppler across the fenestration (if present) measures the 'transpulmonary' PG across the fenestration. If the RAP is known, the atrial pressure can be determined by substracting the mean 'transpulmonary' PG from the RAP.

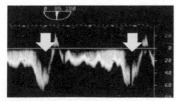

Mechanical versus spontaneous respiration in Fontan circulation: during spontaneous respiration the flow is increased during inspiration. (yellow arrows)

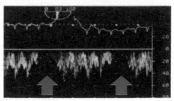

During mechanical positive pressure ventilation the flow is stopped or might be reversed during inspiration. (purple arrows)

TOE sequence for the evaluation of Fontan

1. Look for residual defects like AV valve dysfunction, subaortal or AS, or LVOTO which are all poorly tolerated.
2. Check the flow through fenestration, when present.
3. Exclude stenosis on the Fontan anastomosis.
4. Assess ventricular function.
5. Manage adequate volemia, inotropic stimulation and ventilatory settings.

20.3 References

1. Simpson J, et al. *Three-dimensional echocardiography in congenital heart disease: an expert consensus document from the European Association of Cardiovascular Imaging and the American Society of Echocardiography.* J Am Soc Echocardiogr (2017) 30:1-27.
2. Puchalski MD, et al. *Guidelines for Performing a Comprehensive Transesophageal Echocardiographic Examination in Children and All Patients with Congenital Heart Disease: Recommendations from the American Society of Echocardiography.*
J Am Soc Echocardiogr (2019) 32(2): 173-215.
3. Bettex DA, et al. *Intraoperative transesophageal echocardiography in pediatric congenital heart surgery: A two-center observational study.* Anesth Analg (2003) 97: 1275-82.

21

TOE for Heart Transplants

DONNA GREENHALGH
STEFAAN BOUCHEZ

21.1 Introduction

The number of heart and lung transplantations has risen over the years, and they remain the mainstay of treatment for end-stage heart failure. From the assessment of the donor's heart to intraoperative management during separation from CPB to the postoperative follow-up of heart transplant patients, echocardiography plays a vital role throughout this process.

Donor Hearts
- Braindead heart donors make up the majority of the cardiac donor pool.
- Brain death decreases LV-EF: 'neurogenic stunned myocardium'
  - LV dysfunction is mostly temporary.
  - LV-EF $\geq$ 40 % can safely be transplanted.
- Check for LVH: LV WT $\leq$ 13 mm.
- Congenital laesions: PFO, ASD, etc.
- Valvular pathology.

21.2 Echocardiography

21.2.1 Pre – CPB

Check recipient's heart for:
- Thrombi in LV, RV, atria and LAA. Especially if on mechanical support preoperatively.
- Aortic atheromata.
- Pleural effusions.

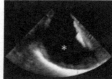
Pleural fluid (yellow asterisk)

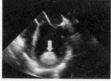
LV apical thrombus (yellow arrow)

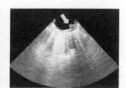
Aortic atheroma (yellow arrow)

De-airing

Adequate de- airing is crucial in heart transplantation.
- Right side: pulmonary air emboli may cause further elevation of PAP.
- Left side: systemic air emboli (brain, RCA) may lead to RV and LV dysfunction, life-threatening arrhythmias, and transient or permanent neurologic deficits.

Left ventricle
- Increased WT: 'pseudo-hypertrophy' related to myocardial ischemia and oedema.
- Systolic function.
  - Related to brain-dead donor, poor myocardial protection, ischemic time, primary graft dysfunction.
  - In normal conditions, LV systolic function appears normal or slightly reduced.
- Diastolic function.
  - Related to ischemic time. Diastolic dysfunction is often present in the early postoperative period but improves occurs over the next 6 weeks after transplantation.
  - Diastolic dysfunction worsens with chronic rejection.
    ○ TDI E/e' ratio < 11: normal prognosis.
    ○ TDI E/e' ratio > 20: poor prognosis.

Right ventricle
- RV function.
  - Related to poor myocardial protection, ischemic time, air in RCA, high PVR.
  - Major determinant of prognosis as it relates to > 50 % of all cardiac complications after heart transplantation.
  - In normal conditions, RV WT and size are increased with normal systolic function.
  - High predictability for the use of nitric oxide (NO).
    ○ TAPSE < 0,64
    ○ RV FAC < 24%

- Interventricular septum: diastolic flattening is present in almost every patient. This IVS flattening decreases over the next few months.

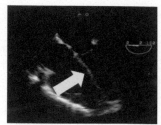

IVS flattening

Anastomoses
- LA anastomosis: a dense ridge with a 'hour-glass' appearance in ME 4C or 2C view.

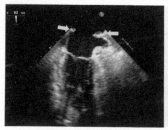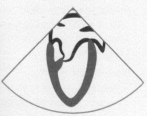

- PA and aorta: both anastomoses appear as a suture ridge ('pseudo-narrowing') in respectively the ME Asc Ao SAX and ME Ao LAX.
  - Doppler velocities aorta < 1,4 m/s and PA < 1 m/s.

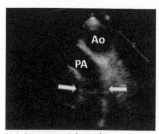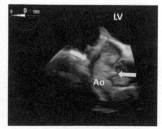

Main PA anastomosis (arrows)   *3D DTG image of Ao anastomosis (arrows)*

- Caval veins:
  - Look for turbulent flow at level of anastomoses.
    - SVC and IVC: ME bicaval view.
    - IVC (hepatic veins): TG IVC LAX.

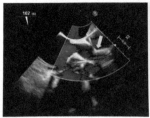 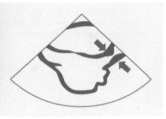

ME bicaval view: anastomosis SVC (arrow).

  - Normal caval flow is biphasic. Loss of the biphasic pattern together with an increase in velocity > 1m/s indicates obstruction.
- Pulmonary vein flow: some difference in the peak flow velocity of the right and left pulmonary veins possibly due to stenosis at the suture line between the LA and right superior pulmonary vein, or compression of the right superior pulmonary vein by the anastomosis between the SVC and RA.
  - Normal PV peak flow velocity < 1 m/s

Valvular pathology
- Mild to moderate TR is the most common single valve disease after heart transplantation and is present in up to 70 % of patients.
  - Related to PAH and RV dilatation.
  - Decreases over the next months to a year.
- Mild MR is present in more than 50 % of patients without major clinical implications.
  - Related to LV dysfunction, bi-atrial enlargement, etc.

21.3 References

1. Tan Z, et al. *Transesophageal Echocardiography in Heart and Lung Transplantation*. J Cardiothorac Vasc Anesth. (2019) 33: 1548-58
2. Badano LP, et al. *European Association of Cardiovascular Imaging/Cardiovascular Imaging Department of the Brazilian Society of Cardiology recommendations for the use of cardiac imaging to assess and follow patients after heart transplantation*. Eur Heart J Cardiovasc Imaging. (2015) 16(9):919-48.

22

TOE for Extracorporeal Membrane Oxygenation

MAURICE HOGAN

22.1 Introduction

Echocardiography is a diagnostic and monitoring tool widely used in all aspects of ECMO support. The pathophysiology of ECMO, and its distinct effects on cardiorespiratory physiology, requires an echocardiographer with high skills to understand the interaction between the ECMO and the patient.

Indications:
- Respiratory failure = VV ECMO as a mode of ventilation.
- Cardiac failure = VA ECMO as circulatory support.
- Cardiac + respiratory failure* = VA ECMO alone or VAV ECMO.

* VA ECMO is usually optimal for pulmonary embolus patients who need ECMO support as it overcomes both the cardiac and respiratory failure.

22.2 Echocardiography

22.2.1 Indications

Echocardiography is the only imaging modality capable of providing real time, point of care, simultaneous structural and functional assessment of the atria, ventricles, valves and great vessels. Next it enables proper visualization and positioning of the cannulas.

RV and LV function
- Biventricular systolic and diastolic function.
  - RWMA.
  - Cardiac morphology: hypertrophic or thin, Takotsubo cardio-myopathy etc.
  - Structural defects: acquired or congenital
    ○ Thrombus.
    ○ Shunts.
- Haemodynamic assessment
  - Quantification of:
    ○ VTI and/or SV.
    ○ Shunt fraction (Qp:Qs).
    ○ PAP, RAP and LAP.

Valvular function
- Secondary changes suggesting acute vs. chronic valvular dys-function: chamber dilatation, ventricular hypertrophy, systolic function etc.
- Vegetations / endocarditis.

Other pathology
Pathology as mechanical causes of shock.
- Pericardial effusion.
- Pulmonary embolus.
- Mechanical complications post myocardial infarction (AMI):
  - PM rupture.
  - VSD.
  - Myocardial rupture.

22.2.3 TOE and cannulation

VA ECMO
- Central ECMO cannulation: drainage cannula in venae cava/ RA, return cannula in ascending aorta, thereby provides mainly antegrade perfusion.
- Peripheral ECMO cannulation: drainage cannula tip in RA via femoral venous access site most commonly, return cannula in descending aorta via femoral artery most commonly, thereby provides mainly retrograde perfusion.

VV ECMO
- Femoral venous drainage cannula and a separate jugular venous return cannula is most conventional.
- Single cannula which incorporates both the drainage and return cannulas in one (eg Avalon®, Protek Duo®) require only one access site, usually the right internal jugular vein.

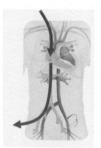 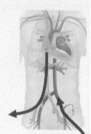 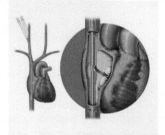

VV-ECMO: femoral venous drainage and jugular venous return and jugular vein return (image by Harvi simulation software).

VA-ECMO: femoral venous drainage and femoral arterial return and jugular vein return (image by Harvi simulation software).

Single jugular venous cannula (drainage and return)

TOE guidance of the drainage cannula

- Both VA and VV ECMO require a drainage cannula, most inserted peripherally via a femoral vein.
- Ideal location for the tip of the drainage cannula for VA ECMO is within the RA or SVC (ME bicaval view).
- Ideal location for the tip of the drainage cannula for VV ECMO is within the IVC, close to its junction with the RA (if the drainage cannula is too close to the return cannula in VV ECMO there is a risk of blood recirculation within the ECMO-circuit).

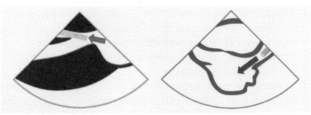

VV-ECMO: Venous drainage cannula in IVC and venous return cannula in SVC.

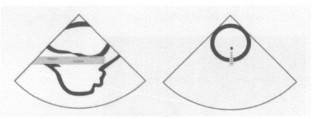

VA-ECMO: Venous drainage cannula in RA (left). Guidewire of aortic cannula in desc. aorta (right).

- Potential hazards of venous cannulation include vascular or cardiac perforation, tamponade, bleeding, or cardiac rupture. These risks can be reduced by cannulating under real time ultrasound guidance (Vascular US and TOE).
- The ME bicaval view is most useful and allows for visualisation of guidewire and cannula placement from either IVC or SVC.

Return cannula- peripheral VA ECMO.

- Most inserted via a femoral artery, usually the cannula is too short to be seen on TOE, however it should be confirmed that the guidewire is safely within the aortic lumen on insertion, and that there has been no dissection after placement.
- Assessment of aortic atherosclerotic disease should also be performed (ME desc aortic SAX and LAX views).

Dual lumen cannula (Avalon®)

- Most inserted via the right internal jugular vein.
- Requires very specific placement and orientation for optimal function, so benefits most from TOE guidance.
- Case reports of cardiac perforation are seemingly more common with dual lumen cannulation than with conventional femoral- jugular cannulation.
- The drainage occurs proximally and distally, with the return orifice in between. Optimal placement locates the cannula tip with distal drainage in the IVC, with proximal drainage from the RA/SVC, and the return orifice directed towards the TV. A modified ME bicaval view allows optimal placement and positioning.

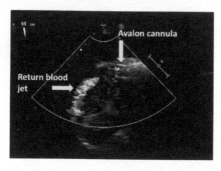

22.2.4 Assessment of cardiac recovery (VA ECMO)/ Weaning from VA ECMO

- Reduce ECMO flow incrementally to 1-1.5L/min only for a brief period (<15 minutes, as the risk of thrombosis increases if flow is reduced).
- Visualize the size and contractility of both LV and RV with echo. Patients whose LV-EF and S wave velocity increase when ECMO flow is reduced are more likely to be weaned. If they remain unchanged, then successful weaning is less likely.
- Reducing ECMO flow increases right ventricular preload. If they RV dilates beyond normal in response to the reduction in flow, then successful weaning is less likely.

Echocardiographic predictors for successful weaning from VA ECMO.
- No important RV or LV distention.
- LV-EF > 20-25%.
- VTI through the AV > 10 cm.
- S wave velocity (S')> 6 cm/s at the lateral MV annulus.
- Increase in LV global longitudinal strain of at least 20%.

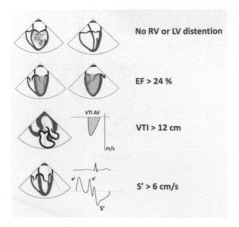

No RV or LV distention

EF > 24 %

VTI AV
m/s
VTI > 12 cm

e'   a'
S'
S' > 6 cm/s

VA ECMO.
- Intracardiac thrombosis – TOE is most sensitive diagnostic test.
- AV opening/native ejection (predisposes to thrombosis if there is intracardiac stasis or non-opening AV).
- Pericardial effusion.
- Air embolism.
- New valvular pathology (most commonly regurgitation).
- Misplaced cannula.
- Cardiac or vascular perforation/tamponade.
- Post decannulation fibrin sheath, or deep venous thrombosis.

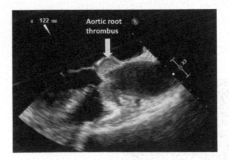

VV ECMO
- Suboptimal position (especially for single, dual lumen cannulation (Avalon®).
- Venous thrombosis.
- PFO or other intra cardiac shunt.

22.3 References.

1. Aissaoui N, et al. *Two-dimensional Strain Rate and Doppler Tissue Myocardial Velocities: Analysis by Echocardiography of Hemodynamic and Functional Changes of the Failed Left Ventricle During Different Degrees of Extracorporeal Life Support*. J Am Soc Echocardiogr (2012) 25(6): 632-40
2. Aissaoui N, et al. *Predictors of Successful Extracorporeal Membrane Oxygenation (ECMO) Weaning After Assistance for Refractory Cardiogenic Shock*. Intensive Care Med. (2011) 37(11): 1738-45

23

Left Ventricular Assist Devices

STEFAAN BOUCHEZ

23.1 Introduction

23.1.1 Definition

A Left Ventricular Assist Device (LVAD) is a device which is implanted through the apex of the LV where it unloads the LV and pumps the blood into the aorta, creating a continuous systemic blood flow (=loss of pulsatility). The goal of the LVAD is to improve *circulatory* output and organ function.

23.1.2 Indications

Patients with end-stage LV failure, as a bridge to transplantation, bridge to recovery or as a bridge to destination.

23.1.3 General considerations

- Surgical correction is warranted in the following conditions:
- Mechanical prosthetic valves (MV or AV)
  - Severe MS.
  - More than mild AR.
  - Severe TR.
  - Presence of an intracardiac shunt: PFO, ASD.
  - Intracardiac thrombus (LV thrombus or LAA thrombus).
- LVAD apparatus has to be considered as a multilayer system.
  - LVAD device has 3 components:
    - Inflow or apical cannula (LV).
    - Outflow cannula (Ascending aorta).
    - The pump or impeller.
  - The LV, surrounding the inflow cannula, serves as a preload reservoir.
  - The RV is the low-limiting pump of the apparatus and acts as the preload source for the LV.

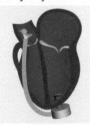

23.2 Echocardiography

23.2.1 LVAD

Inflow or apical cannula
- 2D echocardiography.
  - ME 4C view: In middle of LV, directed towards MV. Avoid oblique position towards LV wall: suction events!

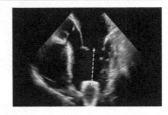

- Colour Flow Doppler.
  - Laminar flow towards apical cannula.
  - The Heartware-system will create an artefact: 'Waterfall artefact'.

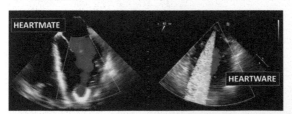

- Spectral Doppler.
  - PW Doppler: 2 velocities, both systolic and diastolic.
    - Systolic velocity = dominant velocity. (< 1,5 m/s). Velocities >1,5 m/s suggest obstruction.
    - A diastolic velocity needs to be present.
    - Measurements not feasible in the Heartware-device (artefacts).

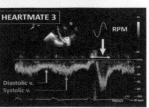

Outflow cannula

- Colour Flow Doppler.
  - ME LAX view, ME AV LAX view to detect the outflow cannula and flow.

- Spectral Doppler.
  - PW Doppler of outflow tract to measure LVAD output:
    - LVAD output = $0{,}785 \times D^2$ cm $\times$ VTI$_{outflow\ tract} \times$ HR
      › D: diameter of outflow tract .
        - Heartware: 1,0 cm.
        - Heartmate II: 1,6 cm.
        - Heartmate III: 1,4 cm.
    - CW Doppler: 2 velocities, both systolic and diastolic.
    - Diastolic = dominant velocity (<2 m/s).
    - See also below (Optimizing circulatory output).

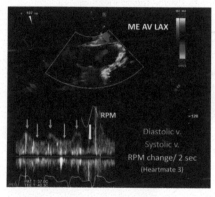

23.2.2 Optimizing circulatory output

- Left ventricle.
  - During unloading LV volume and pressures decrease while aortic pressure increases. 'LV-Aortic uncoupling'.
  - 2D echocardiography.
    - ME 4C view:
      - LV size decreases.
      - IV septum (IVS) position ideally in middle between RV and LV during optimal support.
        - IVS to the right: inadequate unloading
        - IVS to the left: excessive unloading for LV preload
- Mitral valve.
  - Colour Flow Doppler.
    - ME 4C view:
      - Functional MR almost completely disappears during unloading.
      - Significant MR indicates insufficient unloading.
      - MV may remain open during excessive unloading.
- Aortic valve.
  - 2D echocardiography.
    - ME AV LAX: opening of the AV.
      - Optimal: AV opening every 2 – 3 beats during support.
      - Excessive unloading or very poor LV-EF: AV remains closed.
      - Inadequate unloading: AV opens every cycle.
  - Colour Doppler flow
    - ME AV LAX: > mild AR should be addressed during implantation procedure: 'VALVE-VAD' reentry, which leads to decreased systemic flow.

- LVAD outflow CW Doppler:
  - Only systolic velocities: rotational speed is set too low.
  - Only diastolic velocities: rotational speed is set too high for the LV preload present at that time. Caution: only diastolic flow velocities may be seen in presence of hypovolemia and RV failure even at low rotational speed.

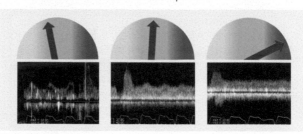

LV unloading overview.

LV unloading	Inadequate	OPTIMAL	Excessive
IVS position			
MR severity			
AV opening			
CWD outflow			

23.2.3 Respect the right ventricle

- RV is the flow limiting pump of the system because the RV serves as the preload source for the LV.
- Incidence of RV failure is high (up to 40%) and 25% of patients needs mechanical support.
- Prediction of RV failure is challenging and depends on
  - Clinical signs, haemodynamic parameters next to echocardiographic evaluation. The correlation between echocardiographic measurements and postoperative acute RV failure remains poor.
  - 2D echocardiography.
    - ME 4C view: ratio of RV/LV ED dimensions.
      - › A ratio < 0,75 is considered important.
    - Functional measurements or poor RV function.
      - › TAPSE (Modified TG RV in and out): < 7,5 mm (nl > 15 mm).
      - › RV FAC: < 24% (nl > 32%).
      - › RV free wall peak longitudinal strain: <- 9,6% (» -10%) (nl – 29%).

FUNCTIONAL MEASUREMENT \ RV/LV RATIO	<0,75	>0,75
TAPSE > 7,5 mm / FAC > 24 % / Strain < -10	proceed	caution
TAPSE < 7,5 mm / FAC < 24 % / Strain > -10	Caution	RVAD ?

- CW Doppler.
  ◦ TR duration corrected for heart rate (TRD$_c$): early systolic pressure equalization between RA and RV because of high RAP and poor RV pressures.

$$TRD_c = \frac{\text{duration of TR signal in ms}}{\sqrt{\text{RR interval sec}}}$$

TRD$_c$ <461 ms: indicates poor RV performance.

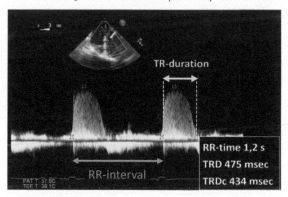

- Tricuspid regurgitation:
  - More than moderate TR impedes RV forward flow.
  - Surgical correction should be considered when TR >2/4 is present together with a dilated TV annulus and a PM/AICD.

LV UNLOADING	INSUFFICIENT	OPTIMAL	EXCESSIVE
IVS position	Rightwards	Central	Leftwards
Mitral regurgitation	Moderate or severe	Minimal or absent	Absent (MV not closing)
CW Doppler outflow tract	Only systolic	Systolic and diastolic	Only diastolic

23.3 The Impella® Catheter.

23.3.1 Definition

A miniaturized ventricular assist device that consists of a pump inserted through the AV and provides continuous drainage of blood from the LV to the ascending aorta. This temporary device (days) is used as a bridge to myocardial recovery, a bridge to a more durable therapy (durable MCS or heart transplantation), or a bridge to decision-making.

23.3.2 Echocardiography.

1. Confirm presence of the guidewire in the descending and the ascending aorta.
2. Confirm the wire crossing the AV into the LV (ME LAX).

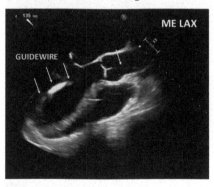

3. Positioning of the Impella® catheter.

The Impella® catheter is introduced over the guidewire into the LV and positioned relative to the AV.

– Optimal positioning of the Impella® catheter.

  ○ The inlet area ('teardrop' appearance in the LV) of the catheter should be about 4 cm below the AV. When the catheter is too deep and touching the LV wall, ventricular arrhythmias may arise.

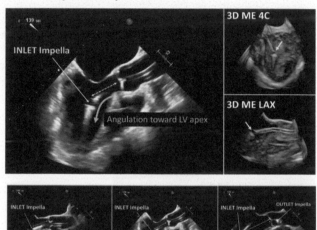

23 Left ventricular assist devices

- The outlet area should be well above the AV in the ascending aorta and is best assessed using CF Doppler. If the outlet is just below the AV, blood will exit the outlet area within the ventricle and circulatory support will not be present.

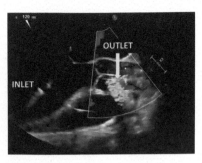

- Interrogation of MV and AV for regurgitation:
  - AR: AV leaflet tethering by the catheter.
  - MR: when catheter is entangled in the papillary muscle and/or subvalvular MV structures.
4. Finally:
  - Assess LV unloading.
  - Evaluate RV function.
  - Check for the presence of 'new' pericardial fluid.

23.4 References

1. Bouchez S, et al. *Haemodynamic management of patients with left ventricular assist devices using echocardiography: the essentials*. Eur. Heart J. Cardiovasc. Imaging (2019) 1;20(4):373-382.
2. Stainback RF, et al. *Echocardiography in the management of patients with left ventricular assist devices: recommendations from the American Society of Echocardiography*. J Am Soc Echocardiogr (2015) 28: 853 – 909.
3. Crowley J. et al. *Transesophageal Echocardiography for Impella Placement and Management*. J Cardiothorac Vasc Anesth (2019) 33(10): 2663-2668.

24

Prosthetic Valves

STEFAAN BOUCHEZ

24.1 Introduction

24.1.1 Types of prosthetic valves

Mechanical valves
Bileaflet:
- Each type has specific flow patterns.
- Comprised of two discs attached to a hinge mechanism.
- When the valve opens, the discs move 80° creating 2 large lateral orifices and a smaller rectangular central orifice.

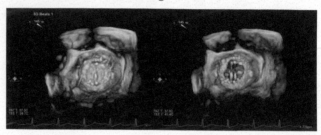

- Retrograde flow across the closing valve consists of 2 components.
  - Closing volume to close the valve.
  - Washing jets: one small central jet and two peripheral jets directed toward the central jet. These jets help to prevent thrombus formation.

Bioprosthetic valves.
- Xenograft (from animals):
  - Stented porcine valves.
  - Stented bovine valves.
    - Advantage stented valves: central blood flow and low thrombogenicity.
  - Stentless porcine.
    - Advantage stentless valves: increased EOA.

- Homograft (from human cadavers): are being used for the following procedures: replacement of AV, TV,PV, MV and aortic root.

24.1.2 Surgical implantation

Selection of the correct valve size
to avoid Patient Prosthesis Mismatch (PPM): the prosthetic EOA needs to be large enough to meet the patient's CO. At the same time, PPM leads to excessive transvalvular gradients.

Orientation of the prosthetic valve
Orientation of the prosthetic valve to ensure optimal valve function and to avoid mechanical complications.

Mitral prosthesis:
- Mechanical: anti-anatomical position to minimize disk entrapment.
- Stented bioprosthesis: avoid LVOTO.

Aortic prosthesis:
- Mechanical: one pivot at the level of the NCC and the other In between the LCC and RCC.
- Stented bioprothesis: avoid coronary blood flow obstruction.

24.2 Echocardiography

24.2.1 Valve seating

Valve seating should be stable and well seated within the native valve annulus. Dehiscence will cause significant paravalvular regurgitation. A rocking motion of the entire valve apparatus indicates significant dehiscence.

24.2.2 Leaflet motion

All leaflets need to open and close normally.
Mitral prosthesis: 2D / 3D using ME 4C, ME LAX view.
Aortic prothesis: 2D / 3D using DTG view, TG LAX.
Optimal 2D assessment of mechanical valves usually needs multiple views as the components of mechanical valves cause acoustic shadowing and reverberations.

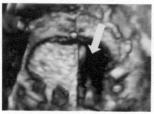

MV prosthesis leaflet dysfunction in 3D: failure to close in systole (arrow).

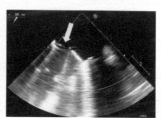

MV prosthesis leaflet dysfunction in 2D: failure to close in systole (arrow).

24.2.3 Regurgitant jets

Transvalvular washing jets
Presence and location of characteristic transvalvular washing jets in mechanical valves at the level of the hinge points. Presence of a small central jet at the level of the coaptation point in bioprosthetic valves and occurs in about 10% of normal bioprosthetic valves.

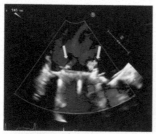

2D MV washing jets (arrows).

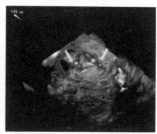

3D MV washing jets (arrows).

Pathologic regurgitation

- Regurgitation within the sewing ring is called transvalvular regurgitation and indicates malfunctioning of the valve leaflets (retained tissue or a misplaced suture interfering with proper leaflet motion).
- Regurgitation outside the sewing ring are called paravalvular regurgitation. Significant paravalvular regurgitation is always pathologic and needs to be addressed by the surgeon. Small paravalvular regurgitant jets (jet area < 3cm^2) will resolve in more than 50% of patients.

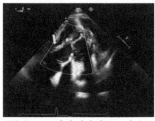

DTG view: paravalvular leak of AV prosthesis.

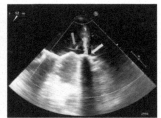

MV prosthetic valve with paravalvular leak (yellow arrow). Normal transvalvular jets (green arrow).

- Generally, the same principles and methods used for quantification of native valvular regurgitation can be used for prosthetic heart valves but are more challenging. A good guideline to grade the severity of paravalvular regurgitation is to measure the VCA and the circumferential extent of the paravalvular regurgitation.

GRADING PARAVALVULAR REGURGITATION	MILD	MODERATE	SEVERE
Vena contracta area (cm^2)	< 0,10	0,10 – 0,29	≥ 0,30
Circumferential extent %	< 10	10 – 29	≥ 30

24.2.4 Adjacent structures

- LVOTO after MV replacement.
- ASD or VSD after MV or AV replacement.
- Coronary artery obstruction/injury.
  - After MV repair or replacement: LV RWMA due to Cx art injury.
  - After AV replacement causing RV or LV dysfunction.
- AR after MV replacement due to misplaced suture.
- MR after AV replacement due to misplaced suture.

24.2.5 Haemodynamic evaluation

Dimensionless Velocity Index (DVI)
AV (peak velocities): $Vmax_{LVOT}/ Vmax_{AV}$
MV (VTI): VTI_{MV}/ VTI_{LVOT}

EOA of the valve using the continuity equation
$EOA = CSA_{LVOT} \times (VTI_{LVOT}/ VTI_{VALVE})$
$CSA_{LVOT} = 0{,}785 \times D_{LVOT}^2$

Prosthetic AS

PARAMETER	NORMAL	POSSIBLE STENOSIS	SIGNIFICANT STENOSIS
Peak velocity m/s	< 3	3 – 4	> 4
Mean gradient mmHg	< 20	20- 35	> 35
DVI	> 0,3	0,3 – 0,25	< 0,25
EOA cm²	> 1,2	1,2 – 0,8	< 0,8
Doppler profile	Early peaking, triangular	Intermediate	Rounded, symmetric contour

Velocity and gradient are affected by concomitant regurgitation.

Prosthetic MS

PARAMETER	NORMAL	POSSIBLE STENOSIS	SIGNIFICANT STENOSIS
Peak velocity m/s	< 2	2 – 2,5	> 2,5
Mean gradient mmHg	< 6	6 – 10	> 10
DVI	< 2,2	2,2 – 2,5	> 2,5
EOA cm^2	> 2	1 – 2	< 1
PHT ms	< 130	130 – 200	> 200

Velocity and gradient are affected by concomitant regurgitation.
Don't use PHT to estimate valve area.
Consider MV prosthetic stenosis when DVI > 2,2 and a PHT > 130 msec are present.

Patient prosthesis mismatch
- Prosthetic valves are inherently stenotic relative to native valves.
- PPM implies the prosthetic EOA is too small for the patients CO needs and will increase transvalvular gradient immediately after implantation or with exercise.
- Clinically important PPM occurs at an indexed EOA: EOA / BSA m^2 patient:
  - AVR: severe PPM < 0,6 cm^2 / m^2 versus no PPM > 0,85 cm^2 / m^2
  - MVR: severe PPM < 0,9 cm^2 / m^2 versus no PPM > 1,2 cm^2 / m^2

Pressure recovery (PR)
- PR is only significant in small aortic prosthetic valves and in aortic diameter < 30 mm.
- PR may cause an unexpectedly high echocardiographic Doppler gradient in a normal functioning valve. Doppler-based measurements detect the peak velocity at the VC and will show a higher gradient and a smaller valve area compared to catheter measurements.

Doppler evaluation of high gradients over prosthetic AV

DOPPLER AV PROSTHETIC VALVE	PR	LVOT OB-STRUCTION	PPM	PROSTHETIC STENOSIS
Peak Aortic jet velocity m/s	> 3			
DVI	> 0,30		< 0,30	
Doppler contour and Acceleration Time in msec	Triangular AT < 100	Rounded AT > 100	Triangular AT < 100	Rounded AT > 100

24.2.6 Late complications after valve replacement

- Degeneration of tissue valves:
  - Cusp thickening and calcification leads to restriction of cusp motion.
  - Leaflet degeneration may lead to cusp tear and valvular regurgitation.
- Thrombosis and pannus:
  - Causes stenosis or obstruction by interference with opening and closure of the prosthetic valve.
- Haemolysis:
  - Associated with severe paravalvular regurgitation.
- Endocarditis:
  - Occurs in 3 % of patients within the first year of implantation with a 1 % annual incidence thereafter.
  - Includes vegetations, annular abscess, new dehiscence and new valvular regurgitation.

Normal reference values of EOA for the prosthetic AV.

AORTIC PROSTHETIC VALVE SIZE	19	21	23	25	27	29
STENTED BIOPROSTHETIC VALVES						
Mosaic	1,1	1,2	1,4	1,7	1,8	2,0
Hancock II	-	1,2	1,3	1,5	1,6	1,6
Carpentier-Edwards Perimount	1,1	1,3	1,5	1,8	2,1	2,2
Carpentier-Edwards Magna	1,3	1,5	1,8	2,1	-	-
Biocor (Epic)	1,0	1,3	1,4	1,9	-	-
Mitroflow	1,1	1,2	1,4	1,6	1,8	-
Trifecta	1,4	1,6	1,8	2,0	2,2	2,4
STENTLESS BIOPROSTHETIC VALVES						
Medtronic Freestyle	1,2	1,4	1,5	2,0	2,3	-
St Jude Medical Toronto SPV	-	1,3	1,5	1,7	2,1	2,7
Prima Edwards	-	1,3	1,6	1,9	-	-
MECHANICAL VALVES						
Medtronic-Hall	1,2	1,3	-	-	-	-
St Jude Medical Standard	1,0	1,4	1,5	2,1	2,7	3,2
St Jude Medical Regent	1,6	2,0	2,2	2,5	3,6	4,4
MCRI On-X	1,5	1,7	2,0	2,4	3,2	3,2
Carbomedics Standard an Top Hat	1,0	1,5	1,7	2,0	2,5	2,6
ATS Medical	1,1	1,6	1,8	1,9	2,3	-

Normal reference values of EOA for the prosthetic MV.

MITRAL PROSTHETIC VALVE SIZE	25	27	29	31	33
STENTED BIOPROSTHETIC VALVES					
Medtronic Mosaic	1,2	1,3	-	-	-
Hancock II	1,0	1,4	1,5	2,1	2,7
Carpentier-Edwards Perimount	1,6	2,0	2,2	2,5	3,6
MECHANICAL VALVES					
St Jude Medical Standard	1,5	1,7	1,8	2,0	2,0
MCRI On-X (*different sewing cuff size*)	2,2	2,2	2,2	2,2	2,2

24.3 References

1. Lancellotti P., et al. *Recommendations for the imaging assessment of prosthetic heart valves: a report from the European Association of Cardiovascular Imaging endorsed by the Chinese Society of Echocardiography, the Inter-American Society of Echocardiography, and the Brazilian Department of Cardiovascular Imaging*, Eur Heart J Cardiovasc Imaging. (2016) 17 (6): 589–590

2. Cheung AT., et al. *Prosthetic valves*, A.C. Perrino Jr and S.T. Reeves (editors), in book: *A practical approach to Transesophageal Echocardiography*, Fourth Edition, Published by Lippincott Williams & Wilkins, Philadelphia, pp 313 – 344.

25

Transcatheter Aortic Valve Replacement (TAVR) / Implantation (TAVI)

MASSIMILIANO MEINERI

25.1 Introduction

Smaller delivery catheters, modern percutaneous arterial access closure devices and experience with trans-catheter valve (TAV) Implantation (TAVI) or Replacement (TAVR) has resulted into the current minimalistic approach. Most procedures, using the trans-femoral approach are currently done under sedation, using the interventional sheaths as invasive monitoring and central venous access. The lack of general anaesthesia has therefore resulted in most center to abandon the use of intraoperative TOE and only rely on fluoroscopy and TTE.

TOE is used when emergent endotracheal intubation is performed, to manage complications or electively for complex implantations or patients' conditions.

25.2 Echocardiography

25.2.1 TTE Examination in TAVR

Intraoperative TTE examination is usually limited to a focused exam post-deployment.

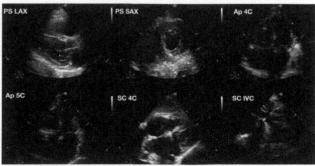

TTE Views PS: Parasternal; LAX: Long Axis; SAX: Short Axis; 4C: Four Chambers; Ap: Apical; 5C: Five Chambers; SC: Subcostal; IVC: Inferior vena cava.

Post-deployment TTE exam:
- TAV position and function.
- TAV Gradient.
- AR.
- LV Function.
- RV Function.
- Pericardial effusion.
- Volume status.

The probe can be left on the sterile field covered with a sheath and used by the interventionalist in case of need during the procedure.

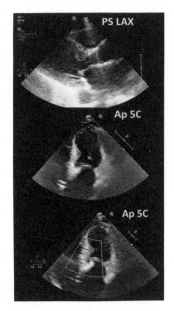

TTE Post Deployment of a Sapien Valve; PS: Parasternal; LAX: Long Axis; Ap: Apical; 5C: Five Chambers.

25.2.2 TOE Examination in TAVR

TAVR can be performed:
- Trans-femoral.
- Trans-apical (through a left lateral thoracotomy).
- Transaortic (through a mini-sternotomy or mini-thoracotomy).

TAVR Implantation consists of four steps:
- Preparation.
- Positioning of guidewires.
- Balloon Valvuloplasty (not always performed).
- Valve Deployment.

Several different valves are currently available. They can be divided into: Self expandable (the stent frame is crimped and dilates once released) and Balloon/Mechanical/Ring expandable (the stent frame is crimped and must be actively dilated). These prostheses can also be re-positionable and/or retrievable.

VALVE TYPE	SELF EXPANDABLE	BALLOON/ MECHANICAL EXPANDABLE	RE-POSITION-ABLE	RETRIEVABLE	SIZES(MM)
Sapien	Yes	No	Yes	No	20-29
Evolut	No	Yes	No	No	23-31
Lotus	No	Yes	Yes	Yes	23-27
Accurate	Yes	No	No	No	23-27
Jena	Yes	No	Yes	No	23-27
Portico	Yes	No	Yes	No	23-25

Preparation for valve delivery consists of the following steps:
- Positioning of pigtail catheters in the aortic root and in the LV.
- Measurement of the transvalvular gradient.
- Positioning of a ventricular wire.
- Positioning of a venous pacemaker (alternatively the ventricular wire can be used for pacing).

Planning for TAVR is typically based on Computer Tomography. When not available TOE can be used for this purpose.

Pre-procedural TOE
- Severity of AS.
- Severity of AR.
- Calcium and Valve morphology.
- Tricuspid vs. BAV.
- AV annulus measurements in 2D and 3D (MPR).
- Height of coronary ostia from annular plane.
- Interventricular septal (IVS) hypertrophy or bulging
- AV-MV annulus angle.
- LV Function.
- RV Function.

- LV RWMA.
- MR.
- Assessment of Aortic Arch and the descending thoracic aorta.

Multiplane or biplane mode can be used from a ME SAX view to position the long axis view to cut through the maximum AV annulus diameter between the NCC and LCC and the middle of the RCC.

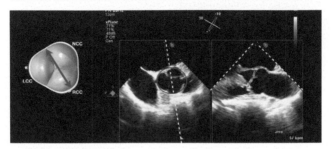

Multiplane mode.
3D MPR of the AV and multiplane imaging significantly increase the accuracy in measuring AV diameter.

A 3D full volume dataset obtained from a ME LAX view is imported into 3D MPR. The Green plane is positioned along the maximum diameter of the AV annulus. The annulus is measured in the green panel that corresponds to the ME LAX view.

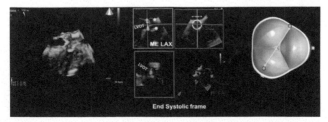

Presence of IVS Hypertrophy specially when localized in the distal LVOT, as well as a narrow MV-AV angle (< 120°) make TAV positioning extremely challenging.

Balloon Valvuloplasty is often performed to increase the valve area and facilitate TAV positioning.

TOE for Balloon Valvuloplasty
- Confirmation that the balloon remains still during inflation (ME AV LAX).
- Rule out complications:
  - Pericardial effusion.
  - Severe AR.
  - LV RWMA.

TOE for valve positioning
ME AV LAX:
- Rule out aortic dissection once the TAV is in the aortic root.
- TAV through the AV annulus.
- TAV height in respect to AV annulus (confirmed by fluoroscopy).
- Correct valve positioning for Sapien and Core-valve.

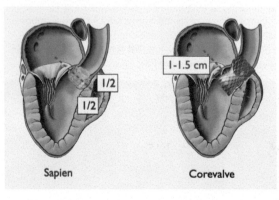

Sapien   Corevalve

TOE Post Deployment
- TAV height in respect to AV annulus.
- TAV leaflet opening.
- AR.
- TAV Gradient.
- LVOT gradient .
- LVOT CF Doppler (laminar vs. turbulent).
- MR.
- Rule out complications:
  – Pericardial effusion.
  – LV RWMA.
  – Valve embolization.
  – Paravalvular leaks.

Quantification of paravalvular leaks benefits from 3D Color display. To minimize shadowing the 3D dataset should be acquired from a DTG view and rotated to a surgical view.
Quantification of paravalvular leaks is based on the % of the TAV circumference involved by the leak:

LEAK % OF CIRCUMFERENCE	AR SEVERITY
< 10	Mild
10-20	Moderate
>20	Severe

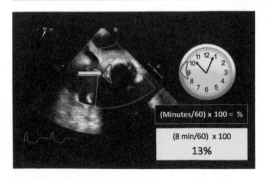

25.3 References

1. Zamorano JL, et al. *EAE/ASE recommendations for the use of echocardiography in new transcatheter interventions for valvular heart disease*. Eur Heart J. (2011) 32(17):2189-2214.
2. Baumgartner H, et al. *Recommendations on the EchocardiographicAssessment of Aortic Valve Stenosis: A Focused Update from the European Association of Cardiovascular Imaging and the American Society of Echocardiography*. J Am Soc Echocardiogr. (2017) 30(4):372-392.

26

Transcatheter Procedures on Mitral Valve and Left Atrial Appendage

JOERG ENDER
STEFAAN BOUCHEZ

26.1 Transcatheter procedures on the Mitral Valve

Edge to edge repair: MitraClip® or PASCAL®- System **MitraClip®**

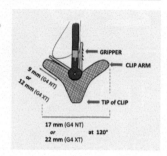

- by far the most common used technique
- with 'Generation 4' four sizes are available:
  - G4 NT, G4 NTW, G4 XT, G4 XTW.
  - The "W" means wider grasping area: 6 vs 4 mm.

PASCAL®

- 2 sizes available: PASCAL® and ACE®

26.1.1 Procedural steps

Start: always perform a comprehensive assessment of the mitral regurgitation (MR) at baseline.

1. Transseptal puncture.
2. "Alignment" or "Clocking".
3. Advancing into the LV.
4. Capture of the leaflets.
5. Control of leaflet insertion.
6. Grading of residual MR.
7. Grading of iatrogenic atrium septum defect (ASD).

1. Transsseptal puncture
Imaging technique:
biplane imaging.

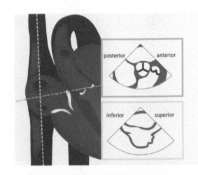

- ME AV SAX biplane: infero-posterior > midline.
- Proper SVC-IVC and anterior-posterior tenting location.

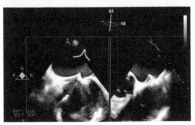

- ME 4C view: approx. 4.5cm ± 0.5cm.
- Confirmation of proper distance from transseptal puncture site to MV annulus level.

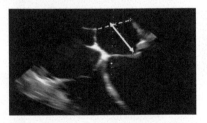

- Biplane from ME bicaval or ME AV SAX at base.
- Puncture and septal crossing (top down "V").

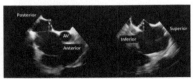

- Modified ME view between 60 and 90°.
- Confirmation of guide wire in left upper pulmonary vein LUPV (white arrow).

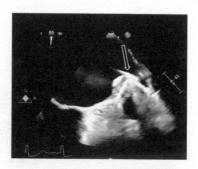

- Introduction of guide in LA.
  - place the cursor on the tip of the guide by using the trackball to visualize the tip of the guide also, in the orthogonal view.
  - avoid too close position to the LA wall.

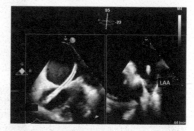

- Introduction of the device
  - MitraClip® through guide.

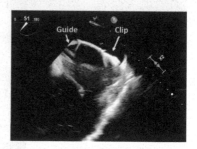

– Unfolded PASCAL® in LA.

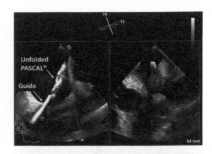

– Folded PASCAL® in LA.

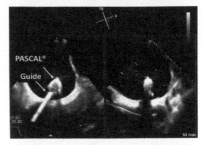

2. **Alignment or clocking.**
Imaging modality: 3D Zoom
from ME bicommissural view.
- Perpendicular orientation of
  the arms to both leaflets.
- 'Clocking' of the device to
  ensure proper orientation.

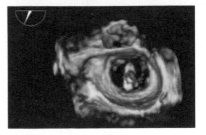

3. Advancing into the ventricle

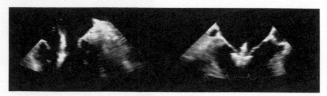

Imaging modality: biplane imaging from ME bicommissural view.
- Biplane: ME bicommissural and ME AV LAX views.
- Ensure non-oblique advancement of the device into LV.
- Check correct alignment to the MV annulus.

- 3D Zoom with reduced gain.
- Check correct alignment or clocking (arrow: indicating the clip).

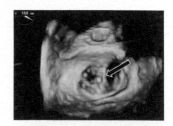

4. Capture of the leaflets
Imaging modality: biplane imaging from ME bicommissural view.
- Ensure that both leaflets run into the device (arrows).
- Record the whole process of grasping the leaflets.
- Use retrospective recording.

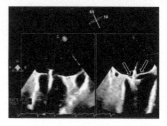

5. Control of leaflet insertion
Imaging modality: 3D Zoom and biplane imaging.

- Ensure that the device creates a broad tissue bridge in 3D tissue bridge (arrow).

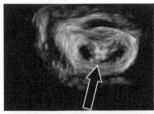

- Control of leaflet insertion: ensure that both leaflets run into the device.

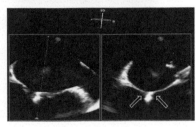

6. Evaluation of MV: residual MR and gradient
Before and after release of the device assessment of residual MR and transmitral PG.

- Grading of **residual MR** is performed according to the published guidelines.
  - 2D: VC width pre- versus post-clipping: reduction > 50% (ideally < 2/4 MR).
  - 3D: VCA.
    - < 0,27 cm² for < moderate MR.
    - Reduction of > 50%.
- Grading of MVA.
  - Planimetry with use of 3D MPR.
  - Ideally total MVA > 2,5 cm².

- Transmitral PG.
  - Mean PG < 5 mmHg.
  - If mean PG < 3 mmHg AND important MR, insert second clip.
  - PW Doppler of pulmonary veins.
    - Systolic over diastolic ratio (S/D) < 0,98 is best predictor for elevated LAP > 20 mmHg.

7. **Grading of iatrogenic ASD**
- Transseptal puncture: usually a residual left to right shunt.
- Significant right to left shunt needs to be closed.

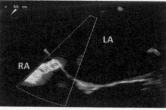

Normal left to right shunt

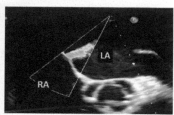

A significant right to left shunt

26.2 Transcatheter procedures on tricuspid valve (TV)

Edge to edge repair: TriClip® or PASCAL®- System.

26.2.1 Procedural steps

Start: always perform a comprehensive assessment of the TR at baseline.

1. Localisation of capture position.
2. Advancing system in RA.
3. Positioning of the device in relationship to TV annulus.
4. Advancing system into RV.

5. Alignment of the clip.
6. Capture of the leaflets.
7. Control of leaflet insertion.
8. Grading of residual TR.

1. Localisation of capture position

Imaging modality: 3D Zoom based on ME RV in-outflow and TG TV basal SAX.

- Visualizing the TV leaflets in 2D: using biplane imaging from the ME RV in-outflow view, sweep from the anteroseptal commissure to the posteroseptal commissure.
- Visualizing the TV leaflets in 3D Zoom, either with the anterior-septal commissure in 5 o´clock or 11 o´clock position (yellow arrow).

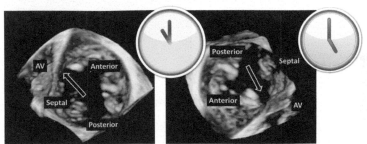

- TG TV basal SAX view Basal SAX view with measurement of the gap at the planned grasping position between septal and anterior leaflet (red double arrow). Use 2D with and without CF Doppler.

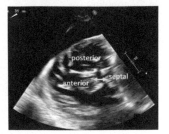

2. Advancing system in RA

Imaging modality: biplane ME bicaval view.

- Visualization of the system in the RA.

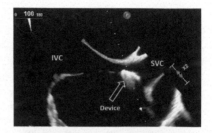

- Visualization of straddling the system to the TV.

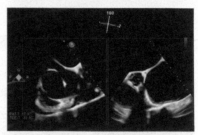

3. Positioning of the device in relationship to TV annulus

Imaging modality: biplane imaging ME RV in-outflow view.

- The device should be positioned perpendicular to the TV annulus in both views.
- Control of independent gripper movement of the device.

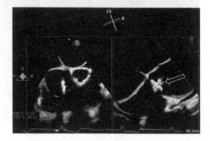

4. Advancing system into RV
Imaging modality: biplane imaging based on ME RV in-outflow view.
- Ensure orthogonal advancement of the device in relation to the TV annulus in both planes.

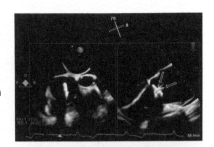

Alignment of clip
Imaging modality: 2D TG TV basal SAX or biplane starting from the TG TV basal SAX.
- Guiding proper localization and alignment of the clip.

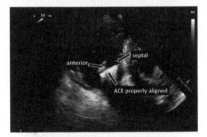

Capture of the leaflets
Imaging modality: biplane imaging ME RV in-outflow view
- Preferred is the ME RV in-outflow view with the cursor positioned at the device.
- Retrospective recording of the capture procedure to ensure that both leaflets are running into the device.
  - Yellow arrow: anterior leaflet.
  - White arrow: septal leaflet.

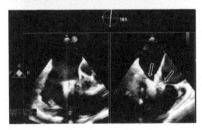

Control of leaflet insertion

Imaging modality: ME RV in-outflow and TG TV basal SAX view

- Look carefully at correct leaflet insertion.
- Use trackball to move the cursor in the position where visualization is best.

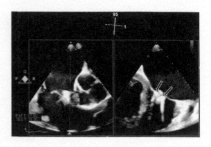

Evaluation of TV: residual TR and gradient

- Grading of **residual TR** is performed according to the published guidelines.
  - Significant reduction in TR jet area (not recommended to grade TR).
  - 2D: VC width, VCA and PISA radius (Nq 30-40 cm/s). PISA measurements are not always feasible in patients with multiple or eccentric residual jets.
  - 3D: VCA.
- Transtricuspid PG.
  - Mean PG < 5 mmHg.

26.3 Left atrial appendage (LAA) closure

Rationale: to reduce the risk of thromboembolism from LAA in patients with non-valvular atrial fibrillation (AF) who cannot tolerate anticoagulants.

26.3.1 Procedural steps for LAA closure

1. Pre-procedural TOE.
2. LAA sizing.
3. Transseptal puncture.
4. Device release criteria (PASS-test).
5. Post-deployment assessment.

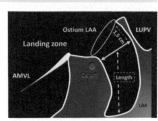

Pre-procedural TOE
- Absence of interatrial shunt, IAS aneurysm or any other device.
- No severe MS or MR.
- No LV thrombus.
- No pericardial effusion.
- No thrombus in LAA.
- Good RV and LV function.
- Identify the LAA anatomy, morphology and surroundings LAA morphology:

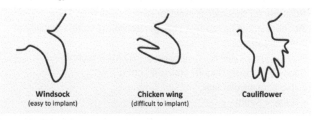

| **Windsock** | **Chicken wing** | **Cauliflower** |
| (easy to implant) | (difficult to implant) | |

- Check pulmonary vein flow velocity: LUPV (to compare post-procedure).

LAA sizing

Haemodynamic goal: keep patient normovolemic and ensure LAP > 10 mmHg.

- 2D ME TOE measurements of LAA diameter at 0°, 45°, 90°, 135°.
- Select largest diameter and depth of LAA at ES (=diastolic for LA).
- Landing zone measurement at level of Cx art. to a point 1 – 2 cm distally from tip of the rim to LUPV.

Transseptal puncture

Technique similar to MV interventions.

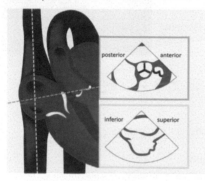

Device release criteria (PASS-test)

Position: no shoulder present or limit to less than 1/3.

Anchoring: tug or tap-test (LAA//watchman) to test stability of implantation.

Size: < 20% of device compression (3D MPR technique).

Seal: CF Doppler Nyquist limit < 40 cm/s.

- No paravalvular leak.
- Leak < 5 mm.

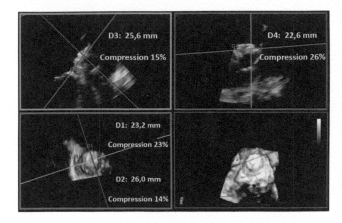

Post-deployment assessment

- Check position of the device using biplane 2D or 3D TOE.
- Assessment of pulmonary vein flow (compare to pre-procedure).
- Evaluate LV function: RWMA (Cx art.).
- Check for presence of pericardial fluid.

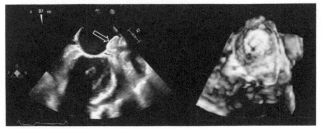

Position of the device after deployment

26.4 References

1. Katz WE, et al. *Echocardiographic evaluation and guidance for MitraClip procedure.* Cardiovasc Diagn Ther. (2017) 7(6):616-632
2. Ro R, et al. *Echocardiographic imaging for transcatheter tricuspid edge-to-edge repair.* J Am Heart Assoc. (2020) 9(5): e015682
3. Agarwal S, et al. *Transesophageal Echocardiographic Guidance in the Implantation of a Watchman Left Atrial Appendage Closure Device.* (2020) 14(11): e01309

27

Perioperative Echocardiography Report

ROBERTO MOSCA

27.1 Introduction

27.1.1 Key points

- General anaesthesia and IPPV create different loading conditions for the heart!
- Blood pressure should be normalized when grading pathology like regurgitation or gradients, under general anaesthesia.
- Be consistent and systematic in your approach. A standard systematic approach ensures complete studies, improves reproducibility and interpretation by other physicians.

27.1.2 Headings

- Patient demographics: name, hospital ID, gender, height and weight (BSA).
- Name of the operator.
- Heart rate, rhythm, blood pressure need to be reported.
- Date, time, and equipment employed.
- Indication for the examination.

27.1.3 Focussed Cardiac Ultrasound or FoCUS

- Point of care cardiac ultrasound examination performed according to a standardized, but restricted scanning protocol to detect a limited number of critical cardiac conditions.
- FoCUS should therefore never be considered as echocardiographic examination. The cardiac ultrasound exam should include
  - Global LV and RV dimensions and function.
  - The presence of pericardial fluid/effusion.
  - Intravascular volume assessment and fluid responsiveness.
  - The identification of valvular abnormalities.

27.2 EACTAIC Perioperative TOE Report

Name _____
Date of birth _____
ID _____

Date: ___/___/___
Elective ☐ Emergency ☐
Age: _____ Height: _____
ECG: SR ☐ AFib ☐ Pacing ☐ CPR ☐

Insertion: Easy / Difficult / Laryngoscopy
Image quality: Good / Moderate / poor
Weight: _____ BSA: _____ m2
HR: _____ BP: _____ mmHg

Surgery: _____

Ventricle	Morphology and vol. status n = normal h = hypertrophied d = dilated	Global function 1 = normal 2 = mildly reduced 3 = moderately reduced 4 = severely reduced	Regional wall motion abnormalities (0 = not scored, 1 = normokinetic, 2 = hypokinetic, 3 = akinetic; 4 = dyskinetic)	Measurements
Left Ventricle				LVIDd _____ (mm) LVIDs _____ (mm) LV-EF _____ (%)
Right Ventricle				TAPSE _____ (mm) FAC _____ (%)

271

ATRIUM	Normal	Dilated	Spontaneous echo contrast	Thrombus (Size, location, appearance)	Tumor (Size, location, appearance)	Device (Size, location, appearance)
Left Atrium						
Right Atrium						

Septum	Normal	Hypertrophied	Shunt	Anomaly (VSD, ASD, PFO, Aneurysm)
IVS				
IAS				

Pericardial effusion (mm): (Loculated /Circumferential):

Pleural effusion (mm): (left/right)

Aorta	Normal	Dilated	Diameter of Aneurysm (mm)	Dissection (Location/ Entry point)	Thickness of plaques (mm)	Mobile Immobile
Ascending						
Arch						
Descending						

Valves	Morphology and mobility of leaflets	Diameter/Distance	Stenosis 0 = none 1 = mild 2 = moderate 3 = severe	Regurgitation 0 = none 1 = mild 2 = moderate 3 = severe

Mitral Valve		Annulus (mm): AML (mm): PML (mm): C-Sept (mm):	PHT (ms): P max/mean (mmHg): MVA (cm²): Grade:	VC (mm): EROA (cm²): Pulmonary veins: (Blunt/Reverse) Grade:
Aortic Valve		Annulus (mm): Sinus (mm): STJ (mm): LVOT (mm):	P max/mean (mmHg): AVA (cm²): a) Planimetry b) Continuity E. VTI- Ratio: Grade:	VC (mm): PHT (ms): Jet/LVOT (%): Grade:
Tricuspid Valve		Annulus (mm):	P max/mean (mmHg): Grade:	VC (mm): SPAP (mmHg): Grade:
Pulmonary Valve			P max/mean (mmHg): Grade:	Jet width (mm): Grade:

Summary of findings:

Signature Supervisor: Signature Echocardiographer:

Postoperative echo examination including any adverse events:

27.2.1 The conclusion of the report

The conclusion is often read first by the intensivists or consulting physicians. It has to be easily understood and should summarize the important issues.

- Identify the abnormality (compared with previous findings)
- Its cause (if identifiable).
- The possible secondary effects.
- Medical advice should be separated from the echocardiographical report.

27.3 References

1. Feneck R, et al. *European Association of Cardiothoracic Anaesthesiologists (EACTA) and the European Association of Echocardiography (EAE) Recommendations for reporting perioperative transoesophageal echo studies.* Eur J Echocardiogr . (2010) 11(5):387-93.
2. Hahn R.T, et al. *Guidelines for performing a comprehensive transesophageal echocardiographic examination: recommendations from the American Society of Echocardiography and the Society of Cardiovascular Anesthesiologists.* J Am Soc Echocardiogr. 2013; 26(9):921-64.
3. Wheeler R, et al. *A minimum dataset for a standard transoesophageal echocardiogram: a guideline protocol from the British Society of Echocardiography.* Echo Research and Practice. (2015) 2(4): G29-G45

Abbreviations

(A)BP	(Arterial) Blood Pressure
2D	Two Dimensional
3D	Three Dimensional
AAD	Annular to Apical Distance
AMM	Anatomical M-Mode
AMVL	Anterior Mitral Valve Leaflet
Ao	Aorta
AR	Aortic Regurgitation
AS	Aortic Stenosis
ASD	Atrial Septum Defect
AV	Aortic Valve
AVA	Aortic Valve Area
AVR	Aortic Valve Replacement
BAV	Bicuspid Aortic Valve
BSA	Body Surface Area
CABG	Coronary Artery Bypasss Grafting or Surgery
CF Doppler	Color Flow Doppler
CL	Coaptation Length
CO	Cardiac Output
CPB	Cardiopulmonary bypass
CRT	Cardiac Resynchronisation Therapy
CS	Coronary Sinus
CSA	Cross Sectional Area
CT	Computer Tomography
CW Doppler	Continuous Wave Doppler
Cx art.	Circumflex Artery
D	Diameter
DBP	Diastolic Blood Pressure
DT	Deceleration Time
DTG	Deep Trangastric
DVI	Dimensionless Velocity Index
ECG	Electrocardiography
ECMO	Extracorporeal Membrane Oxygenation
ED	End-diastolic
EDA	End-diastolic Area

EDV	End-diastolic Volume
EF	Ejection Fraction
EH	Effective Height
EI	Eccentricity Index
EOA	Effective Orifice Area
EROA	Effective Regurgitant Orifice Area
ES	End-systolic
ESA	End-systolic Area
ESV	End-systolic Volume
FAC	Fractional Area of Contraction
FC	Fontan conduit
FS	Fractional Shortening
GI	Gastrointestinal
GLPSS	Global Longitudinal Peak Systolic Strain
HOCM	Hypertrophic Obstructive Cardiomyopathy
HR	Heart Rate
IABP	Intra-Aortic Balloon Pump
IAS	Interatrial Septum
IPPV	Intermittent Positive Pressure Ventilation
IVC	Inferior Vena Cava
IVC-DI	Inferior Vena Cava Distensibility Index
IVS	Interventricular Septum
KPMS	Kissing Papillary Muscle Sign
L	Length
LA	Left Atrium
LAA	Left Atrial Appendage
LAD	Left Anterior Descendens artery
LAP	Left Atrial Pressure
LAX	Long Axis
LCC	Left Coronary Cusp
LV	Left Ventricle
LVAD	Left Ventricular Assist Device
LV EDA	Left Ventricular End-diastolic Area
LV ESA	Left Ventricular End-systolic Area
LVH	Left Ventricular Hypertrophy

LVIDd	Left Ventricular Internal Dimension in diastole
LVIDs	Left Ventrcicular Internal Diameter in systole
LVOT	Left Ventricular Outflow Tract
LVOTO	Left Ventricular Outflow Tract Obstruction
LVP	Left Ventricular Pressure
MAC	Mitral Annular Calcification
MAPSE	Mitral Annular Plane of Excursion
ME	Mid Oesophageal
MLSI	Mitral Valve Separation Index
mPAP	mean Pulmonary Artery Pressure
MPR	Muliplanar Reconstruction
MR	Mitral Regurgitation
MS	Mitral Stenosis
MV	Mitral Valve
MVA	Mitral Valve Area
MVR	Mitral Valve Replacement
NCC	Non Coronary Cusp
NG	Nasogastric
PA	Pulmonary Artery
PACT	pulmonary Acceleration Time
PAH	Pulmonary Arterial Hypertension
PAP	Pulmonary Artery Pressure
PAPVR	Partial Anomalous Pulmonary Venous Return
PASP	Pulmonary Arterial Systolic Pressure
PFO	Patent Foramen Ovale
PG	Pressure Gradient
PHT	Pressure Half Time
PISA	Proximal Isovelocity Surface Area
PLSVC	Persistent Left Superior Vena Cava
PM	Papillary Muscles
PMVL	Posterior Mitral Valve Leaflet
PPM	Patient Prosthesis Mismatch
PR	Pressure Recovery
PV	Pulmonic Valve
PVR	Pulmonary Vascular Resistance

PW Doppler	Pulsed Wave Doppler
Qp	Pulmonary Flow
Qs	Systemic Flow
RA	Right Atrium
RAA	Right Atrial Appendage
RAP	Right Atrial Pressure
RCA	Right Coronary Artery
RCC	Right Coronary Cusp
RV	Right Ventricle
RVD	Right Ventricular Dimension
RV EDA	Right Ventricular End-Diastolic Area
RV ESA	Right Ventricular End-Systolic Area
RVOT	Right Ventricular Outflow Tract
RVOTO	Right Ventricular Outflow Tract Obstruction
RVSP	Right Ventricular Systolic Pressure
RWMA	Regional Wall Motion Abnormalities
SAM	Systolic Anterior Motion of Anterior Mitral Leaflet
SAX	Short Axis
SBP	Systolic Blood Pressure
STJ	Sino-Tubular Junction
SVC	Superior Vena Cava
SVC-CI	Superior Vena Cava Collapsibility Index
SVI	Stroke Volume Index
SVR	Systemic Vascular Resistance
SVS	Sinusses of Valsalva
SVV	Stroke Volume Variation
TA	Tricuspid Annulus
TAPSE	Tricuspid Annular Plane of Excursion
TAVI	Transcatheter Aortic Valve Replacement
TAVR	Transcatheter Aortic Valve Implantation
TDI	Tissue Doppler Imaging
TG	Transgastric
TOE	Transoesophageal Echocardiography
TR	Tricuspid Regurgitation
TRDc	Tricuspid Regurgitation corrected for heartrate

TS	Tricuspid Stenosis
TTE	Transthoracic Echocardiography
TV	Tricuspid Valve
UE	Upper Oesophageal
VA	Ventriculo-Arterial
VAJ	Ventriculo-Arterial Junction
VC	Vena Contracta
Vp	Mitral Propagation Velocity
VSD	Ventricular Septum Defect
VTI	Velocity Time Interval
VV	Veno-Venous
WT	Wall Thickness